CALM

Text © Fearne Cotton 2017
The right of Fearne Cotton to be identified as the author of
this work has been asserted in accordance with the Copyright, Designs and Patents Act 1988.

First published in Great Britain in 2017 by Orion Spring,
an imprint of the Orion Publishing Group Ltd
Carmelite House
50 Victoria Embankment
London EC4Y 0DZ
An Hachette UK Company

1 3 5 7 9 10 8 6 4 2

A CIP catalogue record for this book is available from the
British Library.

ISBN: 9781409176923

Back cover photography: Liam Arthur
Design: HART STUDIO
Black and white illustrations: Fearne Cotton
Chapter illustrations and colour illustrations: Jessica May Underwood
With the exception of the watercolour ripples: HART STUDIO
Activity illustrations: HART STUDIO

The Orion Publishing group's policy is to use papers that are natural, renewable and recyclable and
made from wood grown in sustainable forests. The logging and manufacturing processes are expected
to conform to the environmental regulations of the country of origin.

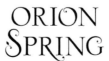

www.orionbooks.co.uk

FEARNE COTTON

CALM

Working through life's daily stresses
to find a peaceful centre

For my husband Jesse,

the calmest person I know

Your
Reflection
Ripples

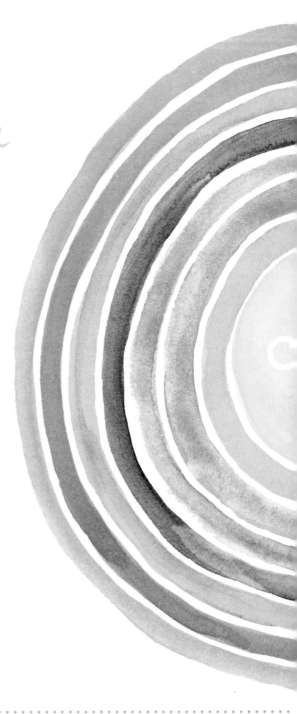

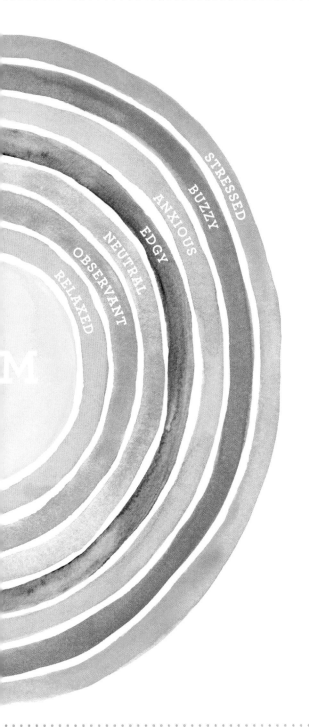

STRESSED
BUZZY
ANXIOUS
EDGY
NEUTRAL
OBSERVANT
RELAXED

M

These are your reflection ripples. As you are reading through the book, whenever you see this symbol:

refer back to this page and mark a dot in the ring that represents how you are feeling. You can then look back and see how you've been feeling over a period of time.

WHAT IS CALM?

Calm is a state of serenity.

Calm is the feeling of being grounded.

Calm is a place we can all come back to if we remember it's there.

Calm is clarity and making decisions confidently.

Calm is remembering there is lots of good in the world as well as bad.

Calm is deep breaths and the feeling of support.

Calm is feeling safe and held.

Calm is accepting it all.

Calm is feeling connected even when everything feels hectic.

Calm is not boring.

Calm is not idle or permanently still.

Calm is not shutting out life.

Calm is not hiding away to avoid the world.

Calm is not ignoring the chaos out there.

Calm is not saying no out of fear.

Calm is not always taking the easy route.

Calm is not forcing yourself to meditate or be still.

Calm is not cutting off roads to excitement.

Calm is not living to the ticking clock.

Calm is not overrated.

Calm is within us all.

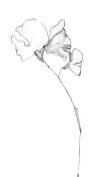

Is it possible to feel calm in this day and age, when we have drifted our focus so far from the basic experience of being 'human'?

How can we feel calm when chaos seems to slip its way through every crack in our personal boundaries?

Is there the time to breathe when we are face to face with work deadlines, children's activity schedules, pressurised social lives and outside expectations that we feel we must fly towards?

I'm breathless just thinking about it.

This is modern life. We are all, on some level, sucked into its messy vortex and churned out the other side with tired eyes, ruffled clothing and many unanswered questions. It may feel like we have to go against the grain in our chaotic, fast-paced modern world to find calm, but it is completely doable. The starting point is realising that we don't have to keep up with the speed of it all, we don't have to facilitate stress every day and we don't have to live up to the expectations of others. Finding calm is a personal project that has to work for YOU!

Whilst writing my previous book, *HAPPY*, I pondered the subject of calm a lot. I thought about its relationship with happiness and how the two states might help each other out. I realised that calm is such an important part of the overall equation if we want to live a happy and peaceful life. It is the nucleus to it all, because if we are calm we have clarity, we can react to situations from a grounded place and we can open our hearts even wider with trust.

The human race has had to take on so much change in the last century. We are constantly on show nowadays, voyeuristically taking snatches of each other's lives;

rushing, pushing, racing and losing ourselves along the way. Technology, the way we view success and what we think we want out of life are all sucking us from our natural roots and catapulting us into a hurricane of sometimes destabilising chaos.

With calm comes contentment, or happiness – or perhaps a bit of both. Or, wait . . . does happiness bring the calm? And are either of these delicious states able to exist without the other? I'm pretty sure that you can feel completely happy yet quite frantic and het up, as I have at many times in my life – those rollercoaster peaks where you could scream because you're so overjoyed. Calm might not be present at all in these moments! I'm also certain that you can feel very calm yet perhaps slightly numb or emotionless at times, too, for instance when life feels slow-paced and uneventful and sits somewhere in the middle. I've experienced these calm moments that aren't necessarily connected to happiness on many occasions.

But I'm also sure that together they can be something quite beautiful, and it doesn't matter if happy brings the calm or vice versa, they are a dual goal to have in mind and they often come in tandem.

I haven't written this book because I have the meditation prowess of a Tibetan monk or because I walk around, peace fingers aloft, smiling serenely at strangers. I've written it because I understand the extreme power and value that calm can bring, and because on a daily basis I endeavour to choose calm over stress. I've written it because at times I feel galaxies away from calm's comforting arms and wonder if I'll ever scramble back to them again. I've written it because it is a state that I'm desperately eager to learn more about. I hope that through being honest with and about myself in this book I can mine a little deeper into calm's riches to benefit myself and hopefully you, too. This book is my way of pondering certain questions that perhaps, deep down, we may all know the answers to already – we just need a little encouragement to remember our own strength in all the madness of the modern world.

Throughout this book there will be interactive moments for you to have your own say on the matter, a chance to take stock of your own life – to write lists, vent and analyse your feelings, and discover more about yourself and your own version of calm. You'll also find some conversations I've had with experts and some wise friends of mine on many calm-related subjects that I've found very useful on this ongoing expedition, and that I hope will be helpful to you, too.

So, first up, do you consider yourself to be a calm person? Personally, I'm not sure which camp I fall into. I'm a hybrid of my parents and a dead 50/50 split of their complex qualities. My mum is a tenacious firefly who is prone to extreme emotions and moving quickly, and from her I get my vivacity and a drive which allows me to get a lot done. My mum combats her perception of outside chaos in the world by creating total order in her life. I have also inherited this need and habit. In contrast, my dad is the 'hour' hand on a clock; ticking much slower than my mum's 'second' hand. From him I get the gift of listening, observing and taking stock, which I can access at the most surprising of times.

So I suppose I'm neither calm nor chaos; I'm all of it. And I expect most of us are like this too, in some measure or another. I've spent the same amount of time meditating and doing yoga as I have hurling short rants of road-rage and throwing inanimate objects at walls in toddler-style tantrums. I believe there is room for all these emotions, but using calm as a base to come back to is imperative. The more I understand the importance of calm for our minds, general wellbeing, relationships and outlook on the world, the more time I spend trying to route back to it.

Some of us might already know our own personal road back to calm – how to breathe deeply when panicked, or can feel completely at peace in rush hour or at a busy train station. I haven't mastered this in all areas of my life yet, but it's something I'm constantly working at and it has become one of my main goals in life in recent years. As birthdays have passed and drama has stampeded through sections of my story, I have recognised how much energy and time I have lost to stress, muddled thoughts and tangled words.

So what is calm to you? For me it's less about thought and much more about feeling. It is a stillness that allows my lungs to expand like hot air balloons. It is an acceptance of the noise around me and having the ability to not label each distraction with a negative or positive. It is seeing the world turning and the chaos entering then departing with an instant acceptance. This doesn't mean that I feel okay about injustice, unbidden drama or negative words, it's just these events give me a chance to feel empathy rather than resentment, have understanding rather than to alienate people, and to learn so much about myself and others. It's a magic alchemy of all of these concepts that might give me a second or even a whole day of 'that' feeling – being relaxed yet aware, still yet dynamic, open yet protected. That, to me, is calm.

It's not always easy to settle into this feeling because sometimes the mind plays tricks on us. As soon as we've felt that first tender touch of calm, the mind whispers, 'Don't forget you haven't paid off that credit card yet, don't get too comfy.'

Then it reminds you, a little louder '. . . And you haven't been to the gym today so perhaps you should worry about that instead of feeling this peace?'

Then, almost shouting, you hear, 'Remember, you haven't achieved half of what you set out to do this month – LAZY.'

There. That delicious glow is now out. The dialogue in your mind has extinguished every last flicker of this peaceful sense of still and has left you needing and wanting something else. What do you do then? I tend to look for a get-out, a distraction that will pull my mind from inner turmoil and allow me to zone out momentarily. Sometimes I'll go for a quick hit from social media which I think might act as a form of harmless escapism, and sometimes this helps, but more often than not it only amplifies what the voices were telling me: photos, reminders and signposts telling me that I'm not enough and haven't done enough. Then I can't relax back into my inner calm.

At times I'll comfort myself with food, as it feels as if that little snack may just fit perfectly into this new-found empty space above my abdomen. At other times I'll get snappy with a loved one because that inner voice and its negative spike has to be released somewhere outside of my own mind. Not cool at all . . .

What I really should be doing, of course, is focusing on that inner orb of light that sits just to the right of my heart, which felt quite warm and comforting only moments ago. Picturing it vividly and knowing it's still there, reminding myself that it wasn't really suffocated and extinguished, and instead my frenzied mind just got distracted and pushed aside that warm feeling.

Calm is omnipresent and ever-glowing, just waiting for us to remember its truth and power. If you want to lock into your own inner calm a little more frequently, or perhaps you feel you have lost the ability to locate it altogether, I hope these pages will act as a map for you to get back home. I'm on this crazy trip with you, also trying to suss it all out, so we can help each other along the way. Even by giving yourself permission to sit, open this book and quietly read is a great start in getting back to that sacred land, so know that you're already well on your way! Let's go hunt some calm together.

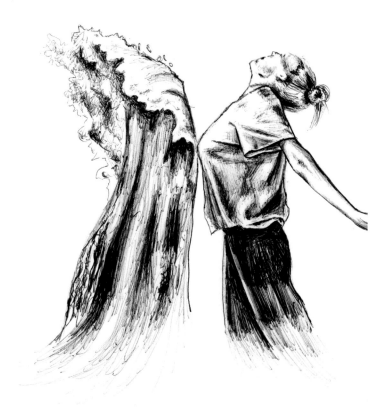

Before we properly begin, take stock of how you are feeling – circle the word that most closely answers the questions below. I find a little self-diagnosis is a helpful way of showing me what needs to change or what I need to work on.

HOW ARE YOUR STRESS LEVELS?	TERRIBLE	BAD	OK	GOOD	GREAT
HOW WELL DID YOU SLEEP LAST NIGHT?	TERRIBLE	BAD	OK	GOOD	GREAT
HOW GOOD ARE YOU AT SPENDING TIME OUTSIDE?	TERRIBLE	BAD	OK	GOOD	GREAT
HOW DO YOU FEEL ABOUT THE AMOUNT OF TIME YOU SPEND ON SOCIAL MEDIA?	TERRIBLE	BAD	OK	GOOD	GREAT
HOW GOOD ARE YOU AT ALLOWING YOURSELF 'ME' TIME?	TERRIBLE	BAD	OK	GOOD	GREAT
HOW DO YOU FEEL RIGHT NOW ABOUT YOUR RELATIONSHIPS?	TERRIBLE	BAD	OK	GOOD	GREAT
HOW DO YOU FEEL ABOUT THE FUTURE?	TERRIBLE	BAD	OK	GOOD	GREAT
HOW DOES YOUR CHEST FEEL RIGHT NOW?	TERRIBLE	BAD	OK	GOOD	GREAT
HOW DOES YOUR BODY FEEL?	TERRIBLE	BAD	OK	GOOD	GREAT
HOW DOES YOUR MIND FEEL?	TERRIBLE	BAD	OK	GOOD	GREAT

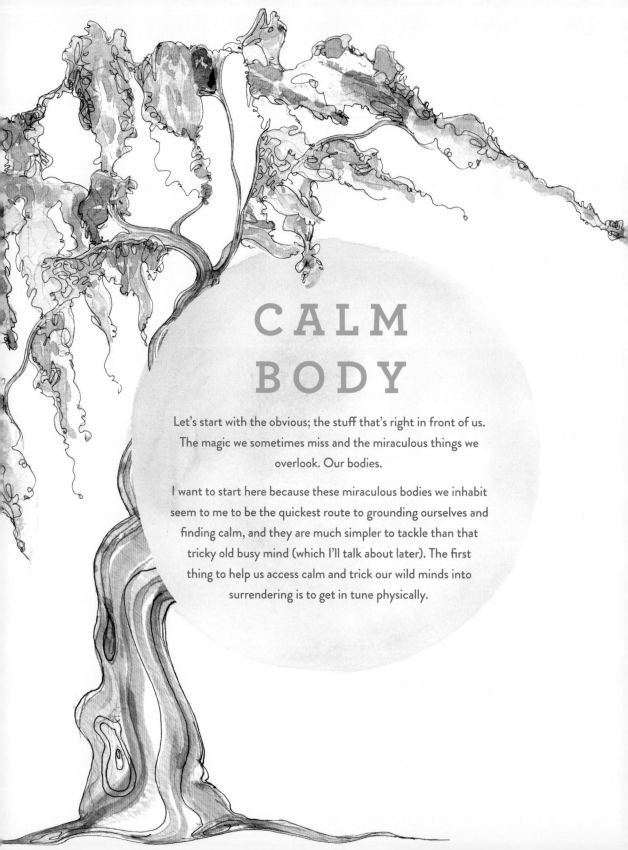

CALM
BODY

Let's start with the obvious; the stuff that's right in front of us.
The magic we sometimes miss and the miraculous things we
overlook. Our bodies.

I want to start here because these miraculous bodies we inhabit
seem to me to be the quickest route to grounding ourselves and
finding calm, and they are much simpler to tackle than that
tricky old busy mind (which I'll talk about later). The first
thing to help us access calm and trick our wild minds into
surrendering is to get in tune physically.

THE SHORTCUT TO CALM

The phenomenal living, breathing, complex bodies we move around with every day are to be admired and cared for. Bones and joints working in harmony to get us moving; nerves and veins facilitating our flow and feelings; muscles and ligaments supporting our skeleton; skin keeping us together, protecting our bodies and allowing us to touch objects or people. When you break it down and remember that amongst all the emotion, thoughts and velocity there is a pumping heart, expansive lungs and millions of intricate happenings inside our bodies, the focus shifts and you can gain perspective.

At times I feel frantic, erratic and foundationless and I can't quite fathom how I will get myself travelling back towards my place of inner calm. It can feel like a vast canyon away, completely concealed in a fog of gratuitous emotions that I can't control. Dealing with my messy brain at moments like this is almost a waste of time. I'll go round in circles and probably get myself into more of a mess by overthinking and analysing the situation. My first stagger in the direction of calm in these moments is purely physical. It is a shortcut that seems almost too easy, but I know it'll work – I've done it millions of times before and I have reaped the benefits again and again.

Only last week I was feeling very uptight and tangled in a story that seemed to be aggravating me on every level. I couldn't make sense of it and I felt suffocated in words like 'WHY?' and 'WHAT IF?' I knew it would be a disaster to try to unpick all of these thoughts and words so instead I threw on a coat and bobble hat and took myself into the early evening air to simply walk. With each step my mind felt clearer. With each new patch of pavement conquered I felt more at ease. With each minute that passed I felt my body surrendering and I knew I was headed in the right direction towards calm. I wasn't walking anywhere in particular or with any purpose, it was more the focus on the physical and the change of pace that lightened my head and shone a light on what was really going on. My worries may not have been completely solved during this dusky ramble but I was certainly in a much calmer place afterwards, and better able to move on to tackle the mental jumble that was unpicking itself upstairs.

For any of you who have read my first book, *HAPPY*, you'll know I have a deep love for yoga. It took me a while to get there with this hobby, but now, further down the line in my practice, I understand the movements and breathing rhythms and where they can take me. I couldn't give a toss about wearing a fancy yoga outfit or having abs of steel; for me it's a quick ascent to a place of total calm, serenity and bliss. Whether I manage all the poses in a class or not, or only do it for 10 minutes in my kitchen, I'll still hit the jackpot every time. The focus on my body and breathing slows everything down and my body likes this very much. After a yoga class I can feel my organs and muscles purring like a smiley gang of cats; cats that have been cared for and nurtured, and so will in turn relax and be content.

Even lying on the floor for five to ten minutes will have this effect on you if you truly let go. Try it. Maybe at the end of a day, in your lunch break or when you have a quiet house, just lie on the floor with your eyes closed and see how quickly your heart rate slows, how your muscles loosen and your nervous system balances out. The brain can only follow suit and match the rest of your body's newfound breezy state, so slow your body down or give it gentle steady movement and everything will seem to align that much quicker.

LETTING YOUR BODY RUN THE SHOW

I learned just how effective this letting go can be when I was in labour with my daughter, Honey. While I was pregnant I had gone on a brief course in hypnobirthing, where breathing and tuning into your physical body is key, so while I was in labour I took in huge long inhales and pushed out deep, earth-shattering exhales and I felt my body calm, meaning my brain did not flip into panic mode; instead it worked with my body, knowing that I was capable and strong. Although intense, there was no sense of fear. It was the best physical experience I've ever had, it felt miraculous and beyond powerful.

With my son, Rex, I hadn't given hypo birthing a single thought as he was my first baby and I was far too overwhelmed with all the other practical details of having a baby, such as 'which baby sling do I buy?' and 'how do I attach a breast pump?'. I assumed the labour bit at the end of the pregnancy would just . . . well . . . happen! Every woman out there will go about preparing for their birth in their own way but because I didn't have the physical tools that I would later learn from with hypnobirthing, I did indeed panic when the time came. For me, the fear was physical, as I had nothing to compare it to. As a result, I endured an angst-ridden labour because my mind was running the show and my body could only experience what my mind was dishing out.

I feel beyond grateful for my two babies and they are the most important thing to me, but their births did teach me the lesson that the state of my physical body can run the show when needed and the 'all talk and no trousers' mind can take a back seat now and then when you really physically let go. What an epiphany for me!

HELLO TO . . . GERAD

Gerad Kite is a dear friend of mine who I regularly talk to for pearls of wisdom and a springboard back to calm. It's dead handy having a mate who is also a 5-element acupuncturist! His connection to calm is crystal clear and his outlook on life is expansive yet grounded.

Acupuncture is very physical and allows the body to rebalance and flow smoothly. Gerad has studied acupuncture for 20 years and understands the balance of the body intricately. His knowledge of Eastern philosophy has always interested me greatly and we often talk about the rhythm of the body and how it relates to the seasons and the ticking of the clock. Here Gezza (as I like to call him) explains the importance of listening to our own bodies and honouring how they want to be treated throughout the day. Getting our bodies in balance is a great way of heading back to calm.

"

The ancient 'Chinese Clock' is based on an understanding of how the energy that fuels us travels around the body and mind over a 24-hour period. There is an amount of energy in every person which comes from the food we eat, the air we breathe and the water we drink. This energy (fuel) travels around the body (much like the blood floods through every cell), flowing in one continuous loop, serving all our organs and functions. Every part of the body and mind is served with this energy at all times, but each organ or function has a two-hour period where it is prioritised over any other and will receive a greater volume of energy during that period to emphasise its task. For example, between the hours of 5 and 7 a.m. the large intestine (colon) is flooded with energy, as this is the optimum time to get rid of the physical – and mental – waste from the previous day. This natural and essential excretion not only cleanses our body and mind but as the increased flow of energy transitions from the large intestine to the stomach, we get the impulse to eat a hearty breakfast and start the day renewed with energy. Conversely, there is a low time for each organ at the opposite side of the 24-hour cycle, and in this example the stomach rests. This is nature telling us to eat less and instead nourish ourselves with good company and fun – the peak time of the 'circulation/sex' function.

When adhered to, this inner intelligence is heath-giving and promotes a great sense of calm in us – providing we pay attention and follow its guidance. Sadly, we tend to plan the activities of our days and nights in our 'heads', making unnatural choices about when to eat, when to rest and when to work, and thus we go against this natural flow. The outcome is a reduction in energy, a disturbance to the natural cycles of sleep, digestion and reproduction and a general sense of malaise – of being out of whack with no apparent cause.

The Chinese Clock is based on the movement of our planet in relation to the sun. It is based on the premise that we have evolved as a species as a direct outcome of this 24-hour cycle. By changing your daily and nightly routine to work with nature rather than against it, you will begin to feel at one with yourself and the world around you and you will enjoy a deep sense of calm.

THE CHINESE CLOCK

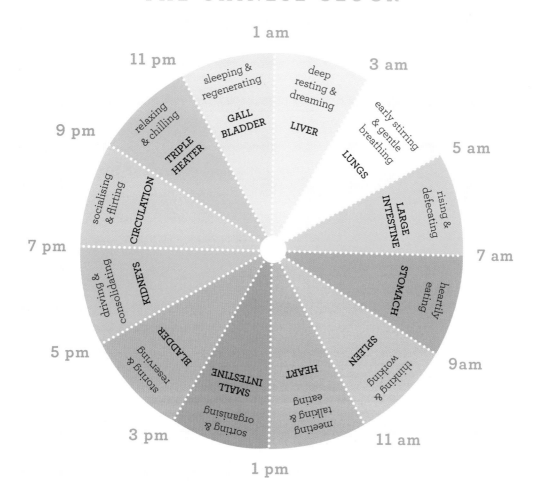

Let's take a closer look at what the clock means for each part of our bodies:

3-5am: your lungs appreciate a surge of energy that awakens all the cells in your body and refreshes your mind.

5-7am: the flow of energy moves to the large intestine, making it the ideal time to wake up and have that bowel movement. This clears out, not just the physical, but also the mental waste leftover from yesterday.

7-9am: During these two hours, the prioritisation moves to our stomachs. Always keep the phrase 'nature abhors a vacuum' in your mind: you've emptied the lower part of your digestive system and now you need to refill so that you have enough energy to get you through the day.

9-11am: The spleen is the focus during these two hours and it transforms what you've taken in and delivers that energy to nourish and move your body and your mind.

11am-1pm: Your heart benefits from a surge in energy during these two hours, so take the opportunity to relax and spend time with other people – socialising, yes, but also the ideal time for friendly, constructive work meetings.

1-3pm: As the small intestine takes its prime time to work, it begins sorting and filtering, so mirror this in your day: use it to focus and organise.

3-5pm: Now the bladder takes over. Most of us see the bladder as being just a sack for urine, but in Chinese medicine your bladder is in charge of your energy reserves, like a reservoir. Make sure you drink enough water throughout the day, so that when you get to the time of the day most known for that midday slump, you'll have enough energy to keep going.

5-7pm: The energy flows through to your kidneys at this time, cleaning out the mind and body: a real opportunity to feel calm and settle from within.

7-9pm: This is the time for your 'heart protector': your circulation and sex facilitators – the optimum time for socialising, relaxing and sex. Avoid that big evening meal and enjoy yourself – this is the stomach's resting time.

9-11pm: The energy now travels to your 'three heater', which adjusts all parts of your body and mind to the correct physical and emotional temperature for winding down after the long day so that you're 'chilled' and in the best state for sleep.

11pm-1am: As we reach the end of the day, the gall bladder comes to the fore. This organ excels in 'judgement' and directs the regeneration of your body and mind, the perfect time to rest and sleep.

1-3am: During this time, the energy shifts to the liver, cleansing our bodies and minds to help us sleep deeply ready for the next day.

What I love about the law of midday-midnight, is the natural intelligence at play that keeps us calm despite how busy our bodies and minds can be. If we work with these natural laws, everything naturally falls into place – we feel calm and life, although busy, is no longer experienced as struggle.

"

TUNE INTO YOUR BODY

Have you ever taken an inventory of your physical self? I mean, just sat and scanned over your whole being, noting what feels good and what doesn't. As I sit at my kitchen table now I can feel, very clearly, the bits of me that are content and relaxed and the bits of me that hold tension and stress. My shoulders are tight and tired from carrying kids and leaning over a laptop. My tummy feels full and content from the dinner I've just eaten. My eyes feel a little sore from lack of sleep and my skin slightly taut, which makes me think I'm probably a tad dehydrated. Doing this kind of body register when you get a short moment of peace and quiet is a good idea. Ask yourself, how is your body really feeling? Where do you store your tension and worry? Does it affect your stomach and digestive system? Your back and shoulders? Your skin? Each of us will have bespoke weaknesses that spark up whenever we are run down or pushing ourselves too hard.

At times I get headaches when I'm mentally trying to accomplish too much and I usually suffer with a grouchy back – not just from carrying the small people around, but because it's where I hold my tension. Worries and fears will cling on to my collar bone and neck muscles and pitch up camp for a while, tightening their ropes and tension the more my brain whirs.

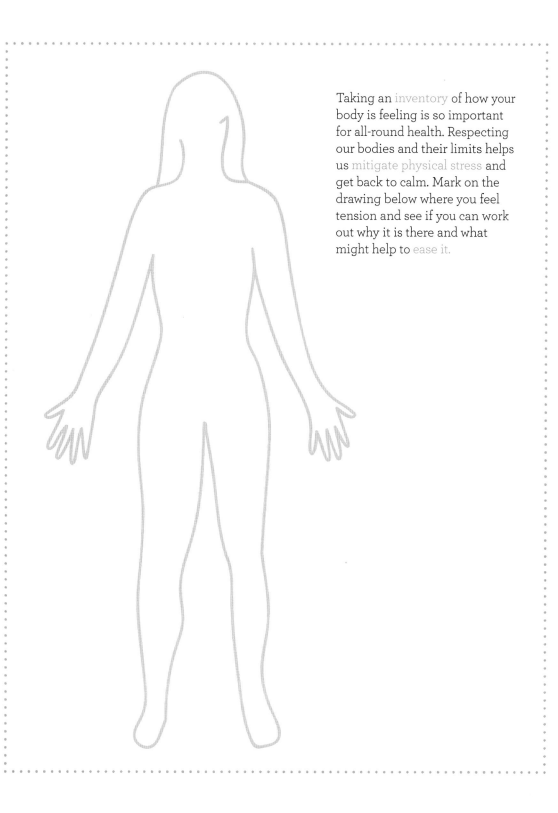

Taking an inventory of how your body is feeling is so important for all-round health. Respecting our bodies and their limits helps us mitigate physical stress and get back to calm. Mark on the drawing below where you feel tension and see if you can work out why it is there and what might help to ease it.

WARNING SIGNS

These are all signs – BIG warning signs – for us to take notice of. This is why the body is so bloody clever; it tries to make it as easy as possible for us to see when we need to change patterns of thought or lifestyle to keep it healthy.

Of course, we all ignore these signs or sometimes don't even notice them as life rockets past at the speed of light. It could be as simple as getting spots on your face, or a recurring pain in your gut, but whatever the physical ailment, it is a sign that the body isn't happy and wants you to notice. Making time to check in with our bodies is vital to support our general wellbeing. We all need to get out of our heads and into our bodies more often.

After the release of *HAPPY*, something rather strange happened to me. In the book I wrote a short piece about anxiety and stated that it hadn't been something that had caused me much grief in life. I always felt that depression was my weakness, but then one day I was driving down the M4 with a great friend of mine, Clare, on a relatively long journey. We were gossiping away about our favourite subjects – the Royal family and *Girls*, the TV show – when I felt rather hot. I opened the windows and wriggled out of my jacket without mentioning anything to Clare. (She herself experienced a pretty bad car incident many years ago which makes me extra cautious when driving her about.) Next my lungs started pumping like a pair of bagpipes. Uncontrollable, short breaths flew out of my panting mouth as the world around me started to spin. This is not exactly ideal when driving at 70mph on a very busy motorway, so I managed to pull over safely and explain to Clare why our conversation about Prince Harry had come to an abrupt end and why we were now on the hard shoulder half an hour from home. I felt totally spun out and discombobulated. What was going on? I have always assumed that personally my physical state comes from direct thoughts. If I think of something negative, my body tenses. If I feel stressed, my body is twitchy. If I feel sad, my body softens. But this was the antithesis of that. Our conversation in the car had been jolly and upbeat and I was on the way home to see my gorgeous babies. No stress, no mental drama, yet my body had taken a turn for the worse. I'd had a panic attack.

I had never experienced this physical manifestation before, so I had no reference to grab hold of. All I know is that it felt like my very soul had jumped out of my physical body; it had leapt out of my skin and was hovering, ghost-like, above me, creating a separateness and intensity. My heart was beating for the two 'me's that were now in the car and my eyes were desperately trying to focus for both of us. It was vastly different to what I had imagined. I've felt panicky and a little short of breath before but this was potent and physically debilitating.

Embarrassingly yet thankfully, I was driven home by the AA that day (thank you, lovely AA man, who also pulled over to let me wee in a pub due to the time it took to get home!) and when I arrived home I sank into a strange mood of confusion. After several hours of pondering and trying to understand why my body decided to shout so loudly that it wasn't happy, I sussed it. I know many people out there struggle with panic attacks on a much more long-term basis and the reasons and catalysts for this differ greatly (see overleaf for a chat with Dr Annette about this), but for me I was simply exhausted. My mind has a habit of telling me to keep going, keep pushing, keep trying, so I do, but now I was discovering I had pushed it too far and my body was screaming out for attention. I'm not naturally good at relaxing so I do way too much most of the time. I love being a mum and a wife, I adore my job and I want to learn as much as I can, but all this leaves no time at all for self-care (more on this in the next chapter). This motorway saga printed out some new rules in black and white for me: NO MORE RUSHING AROUND LIKE A LUNATIC!

I took this experience as a one-off but unfortunately the very same thing happened again, just a week after. This time it was brought on by the fear of what MIGHT happen. Thankfully, though, after a few months of on/off panics I started to find the fear dissipating. Now I can drive without feeling scared, just as I had done for so many years before this incident, and I feel at peace with it all. A hangover of fear has festered to some extent, but I have also pragmatically reasoned with these worries and diluted them so that they stay in the past where they belong. More importantly I've become much more aware of how much I physically push myself.

I know that my brain is often the messiest part of me, so short-cutting to physical tools is my free pass to calm. Breathing deeply, relaxing my body and calming my nervous system will keep me travelling in the right direction to calm. It is imperative that we have some mental space without thought and this is often more easily achieved with some physical activity.

The lesson I learned here BIG time is to listen to your body. If it seems unhappy, if it is throwing you obvious signs, LISTEN to it! Maybe you too need to make tweaks to approach life in a calmer way. I'm sure this applies to most of us out there as we chase hundreds of goals, desires and dreams, but remember that calm is still attainable alongside these ambitions with a little thought and a lot of self-care.

HELLO TO . . . ANNETTE

Annette Twigg is a GP who has advised many people who have experienced panic attacks. After I was consumed by that oxygen-gobbling fear on the motorway, the first thing I wanted to do was understand physically what on earth was going on with me. I love to look outside of the box and figure out new ways of thinking and living, but learning about the medical reasons felt imperative to truly understand how to stop them. Here Annette describes a little more about what happens to our bodies during this process.

F: Hi Annette. Can you tell us a bit about what a panic attack actually is and why some people experience them?

A: 'Panic' symptoms arise out of our response to a threat or stress, and form the basis of the fright-flight-fight response. In such a situation, our eyes pick up on a visual threat and relay the information to the brain, which triggers a chemical response, involving the release of stress hormones, which in turn cause a number of physiological effects. The purpose of these is to increase the blood supply to our muscles so that we can run away from the threat, defend ourselves or indeed attack the threat.

As a result our heart rate increases, as do our blood pressure and breathing rates in order to maximise the oxygen and energy (glucose) levels directed to our muscles, all in order for us to run away. Hence you experience a racing heart, rapid breathing etc.

Since blood is being diverted to the muscles, less flows to non-essential areas – those deemed less important in the response to a threat – such as the skin. As such the skin may look pale, feel clammy and have a prickling sensation, because sweat is released to help cool the muscles. The mouth might also feel dry because body fluid is kept in the circulatory system to keep the supply of oxygen and glucose going to the muscles.

Other symptoms can occur too, such as feelings of loss of control, difficulty swallowing or feeling you have a lump in your throat and poor sleep (because your body is maintaining a high state of alertness). For many people the net result of all this is the sensation of fear, i.e. panic. For others, though, the net result may be aggression or an angry outburst.

A person's individual response to this depends on lots of factors, including coping strategies, previous exposure and build-up of resilience. In day-to-day life the 'threat' we see may be people, places, situations, spiders, dogs or insects, or often it can be the build-up of pressure caused by other people's expectations of us and our desire not to let others down, be that family, friends, work etc.

The important thing is to understand that the physical symptoms are not representative of something that will do us harm, even though they can be very distressing and at times disabling.

F: Have you seen a rise in people coming to you with these symptoms?

A: I believe that current daily lifestyles almost certainly contribute to more people experiencing these symptoms, as we're not very good at allowing quiet and non-stimulation time for the brain nowadays, which is not good for us. But there is more openness about anxiety and mental health now, which is almost certainly beneficial and means people feel able to go to the doctor about it.

F: What can people do if they're experiencing panic attacks?

A: Anything that reduces your overall level of anxiety will also help to reduce specific fears or triggers, to an extent. For example, someone having hypnotherapy for a fear of heights may find they are no longer as afraid of spiders, snakes etc.

Sleep is another big issue with anxiety and panic, and it relates more to generalised stress. Essentially we have episodes of deep (restorative) sleep and lighter sleep, often called rapid eye movement (REM) sleep, during which we may dream or feel we are sort of asleep but our minds are ticking over and thinking of many things which seem really important at the time but in the morning are not so bad. We have to have the correct balance of these types of sleep in order to function.

If we are anxious or stressed/having panic attacks, we often find ourselves going over and over things (this is called rumination). If we are doing this during the day our brains continue with this overnight, so our sleep becomes dominated by REM sleep, which is less restorative and consequently we feel more tired and over time we feel less able to cope, our perspective on life changes, our mood can fall and we end up in a vicious circle as this further impairs our sleep.

Breaking this cycle can be initiated by having periods where we don't allow this rumination. This is the basis for using breathing techniques and mindfulness. Physical activity also helps, as long as we are not thinking. So playing football, doing Zumba or playing tennis etc. is good. At home I tend to say a treadmill is better than an exercise bike simply because on a bike you can pedal but still think, whereas on a treadmill you have to focus more on the activity otherwise you risk falling off the machine.

F: Do you have any final top tips?

A: Whenever someone comes to see me and we have talked through their issue, usually one of their biggest problems is the feeling of loss of control. I try to really reinforce that recognising there is an issue is the starting point and that making an appointment IS them taking control – and that is really important. Without wishing to sound anti-social-media, a lot of people who use it get bogged down with everyone else's positive posts and as such feel that they are the only one feeling as they do. This is something that has to be addressed. There was a lovely phrase in a book I am reading which referred to someone's house not having the 'tinnitus of technology', i.e. no computer, TV etc. I thought this comment captured quite nicely that we do need that space to be free of extraneous 'noise'.

But finally, if you have any of these symptoms I've mentioned here, then definitely report them to your GP if they become distressing. There is lots that can be done to manage them.

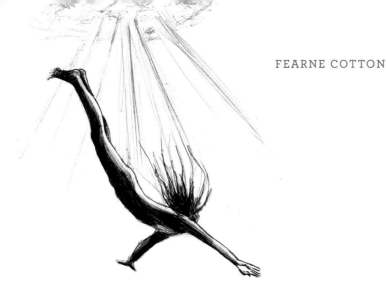

FUEL YOUR BODY

How does stress affect your eating habits? Do you treat your body like a bin, throwing whatever comes to hand down into its depths, hoping it'll fill the holes caused by life's anxieties? Or does your stomach contract into a tiny ball, refusing any bulk or comfort in these times of stress? I think I do both, which is ironic really, as it's the time that our bodies really need thoughtful fuel inside them.

My own stress can arrive in many forms. Sometimes the small daily stresses of keeping the family running smoothly alongside my strange and varied career means that I subconsciously slip into adrenaline mode and feel only the need for nibbles of food and giant cups of coffee to keep me going. At other times, when stress makes me feel low, vibrating and heavy, I may stand at an open cupboard popping snacks into my mouth until I realise no happiness or calm is coming from this particular stint of comfort eating.

Neither of these responses are great for all-round wellbeing, and I think these strange stress- or anxiety-related eating habits are formed when our brains aren't properly 'on'

We hear the phrase 'mindful' thrown around a lot these days, and there is a lot of confusion as to what it really is. One of my great friends, Zephyr Wildman, prefers to use the term 'awake-fullness'. For her, it's about being aware and awake to what you are actually doing. Rather than going through the motions, slipping into habitual behaviour or ignoring the obvious, we must wake up to the reality of what is happening, and if possible route back to the 'whys' of the situation. With regards to eating, being 'wakeful' in these moments allows us to stop and work out if comfort eating or reducing our intake of food is going to lead us down a positive pathway to calm. Of course, there are the obvious things to point out on this subject; if you are hungry . . . eat; if you are full up . . . you may not want to.

Now we've got that out of the way, let's talk more about this thoughtless way of consuming which we know is unrelated to hunger. If you recognise either of my aforementioned eating patterns, look at the after effects of these moments. From my point of view, I can often feel a bit guilty and regretful once I've finished half a packet of biscuits that I didn't really want in the first place. When my stomach is refusing food, I can feel a bit agitated. Yet if our bodies are firing on full cylinders our heads have more of a chance of catching up with the all-round health that our physical body is promoting.

Since picking up on these patterns, I've tried to look at how I can make changes around the times of stress so that my body can be at its optimum even if my head has other problems to deal with. The first step is acknowledging that it's happening, then I can take a deeper look at 'why' and perhaps think again. Do I really want another slab of cheese covered in pickle eaten directly off the knife with the fridge door open and a full stomach, or is it a good idea to push away the plate when my body is crying out for self-care? Once we have awoken to these patterns we can try to act from a place of self-love. If you truly love yourself and want to care for your body, what decision would you make? This is what I try to do each time I know I'm eating alongside stress. Once this physical care is in place we can slowly trot back to a calmer place within.

Being completely realistic, there will most definitely be times for all of us when we comfort eat or eat too little when anxious, so we mustn't beat ourselves up if it happens again – we just need to try and be awake in the moment and reroute back to why we are doing it. Small changes lead to greater ones and are surely a good starting point in getting back on the path to calm. Just remember to fuel your body accordingly. If you are buzzing with energy and ideas, fuel your body to help you achieve what's in your head. If you are feeling low and lethargic, feed your body with some much-needed nourishment. Enjoy each bite and know it's helping you in so many ways. Love the food you eat and it'll love you back.

Cooking and eating can actually be one of the most mindful activities to practise. Luckily I adore cooking, so I can happily canter through hours of the clock, whisk in hand. I love to chop, grate, stir and knead as it stops my ever-rambling inner dialogue and allows me to fully tune in to the physical. I love the rhythm and intricacies of cooking and baking – and I enjoy eating it that bit more afterwards knowing that I've poured time and love into a dish, so I savour the flavour and texture. When I try to finish emails on my laptop whilst eating a rushed lunch or attempt to eat whilst standing up cooking my kids' meal, I feel lousy. I barely remember eating the aforementioned food and it feels almost stuck in my chest area. It can be hard to find proper time to sit and enjoy food in this crazy modern world but try to make it a priority when you can. Small changes in this department create huge ones physically.

Stress is like a snowball – if you don't stop it from building when you first notice it, it will continue to roll and get bigger as it goes. Pick something from the suggested list to stop the stress from gaining any more momentum.

CALM

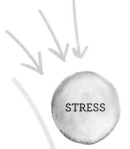

STRESS

Have a bath

Go for a walk

Sit next to an open window for five minutes

Listen to your favourite song (and don't do anything else)

Do one of the breathing exercises on page 65

Close your eyes and think of a calm view

Hug someone

Listen to a guided meditation online

Cover a sheet of paper with doodles

MOVE YOUR BODY

I have always got a huge kick out of exercise. I've tried it all. I'm no Frank Lampard, I can just about kick a football and am probably the worst tennis player to have graced planet Earth, but I love to move. Exercise, to me, has never been about six packs and expensive gym memberships, it's simply about aligning my head and pumping heart and grabbing as many released endorphins as I can get my sweaty hands on. It is instant calm. Moving my body instantly pulls the drawbridge up on my whirring mind; it has no time or space to carry on chattering away as it must concentrate on the physical movement at hand. That instant inner silence is my calm, it's the space that lies between the bubbling pot of problems that I think I have and complete stillness. That space in the middle is where every thought and concern is silently processed whilst my blood pumps around my veins. It's a space where I can deeply route back to knowing I'm okay, and if I know I'm okay, I am calm.

The activities I do can differ and I'm not bothered about the outcome – it could be a run than felt laboured at first but turns into a good 30-minute jog, or an overenthusiastic sprint that turns into a slow walk. As long as I'm moving and my brain is quietening down, the rest is irrelevant.

As well as instantly reaping the benefits of exercise I know that these moments of movement are benefiting my levels of calm in the long term, too. If I'm walking, running, swimming, doing yoga or dancing round my kitchen to Justin Timberlake with the kids, my heart health is strengthening, my cardiovascular system is improving and my general wellbeing is being topped up. I rarely exercise to push myself to unrealistic boundaries as I have no inclination to stress out my body. I have done a few fun stunts in the past, scaling mountains and undertaking long bike rides, but these days I much prefer seeking out physical activities that will benefit my physical state in every possible way. There are so many contradictory statements batted about these days that confuse us further and take away our calmness around exercise, as well as new fads and crazes that we are told we should all try. There are phrases like 'strong not skinny' written in ink; or toned, tanned bodies bursting off Instagram accounts. We no longer know which type of Zumba-Pilates we should be signing up for and what sized calf muscles are seemingly appropriate.

I believe that none of this is relevant; we should all just be aiming to feel good. If running makes you feel pumped and free, then run, Forrest, RUN! If walking your dog feels like a good physical workout and leads you to calm, grab that lead. Just go with what feels good to you. Be strong, skinny, curvaceous, toned, lean, perfectly plump, waify, whatever . . . as long as you feel healthy and full of beans. Good energy equals a calmer mind and surely that is worth lusting after!

My own bespoke routine consists of . . . no consistency. Some days I might run in the park, looking at the ever-changing trees and sunrise on a misty morning. Other days I might have time to sign up to a local yoga class, or I might take the kids out for a walk or bike ride in the park to fill their lungs with air and our heads with space. Do what makes you FEEL good. That'll always lead you back to calm!

THE GOOD STUFF

Sleep. Ahhh, that precious comfort we slip into when the birds stop singing and the black velvet drape dresses the sky. When sleep is good it's orgasmic, but when it's bad it is pretty close to torture. I have bouts of bad sleep, especially since I've had kids. At one point I saw it as more of a luxury than a necessity, a bad habit to get into if you want to stay sane and not look 90 when you're actually 35. Many parents out there will have drifted far from their normal sleep patterns after months on end of breast feeding, changing nappies and generally checking that your kid is still breathing by hovering over them and staring up their tiny nostrils. Even when they learn to sleep through the night you don't feel you can truly let go and drift off with abandon because one half of you is still on alert. People who work nights or have irregular working hours will have experienced something very similar, always awaiting the impending doom of your alarm or a noise in the street which will cause you to wake from a daytime nap.

Lack of sleep most definitely leads to lack of calm. Everything feels weird when you don't get a good solid night's kip. Your focus is slightly off, your concentration is that of a puppy, and your patience and general tolerance of anything and anyone in life is at zero. When I'm exhausted and have had broken sleep I feel like I've gone a bit mad. Nothing seems to really make sense and decision-making is agony. I have been known to stand at a coffee-shop counter deliberating over whether to order coffee or tea for a good few minutes before being forced to come to a conclusion by a very bored friend. Small decisions seem impossible and big ones are completely excruciating. We all need sleep – and of the quality variety. It's imperative to function well in the day and do all we want and need to when the sun is up.

I'm naturally a morning person; I love to step into a new day with a fresh head and new ideas and leap into whatever adventure may be awaiting me. Obviously some days I do this with slightly less enthusiasm, but on a good day I'm raring to go. By the evening my body and mind are both sloping off in the direction of bed pretty early. I can sense the inner need to recharge and recalibrate for the next day's chaos. I love the odd night out but I'm generally shattered from doing way too much in the day. One bad habit I got into last year was going to bed too early. Is there such a thing you ask? YES! I was throwing my whole mojo off by hitting the sack around 9p.m. to read for an hour and then fall into a deep shattered sleep for the first portion of the night. I know, no cool points for this admission! Then the postnatal incontinence would kick in and I was up and down to the toilet several times before the sun came up, which was both annoying and catastrophic for the next day's family time or work.

I was complaining about my broken sleep to a friend who mentioned sleep hygiene. My first defence was to protest that my bed sheets were completely clean and I was fine in that department, but he went on to explain what the phrase really means and how it could help me. The concept was introduced in the 1970s and is a set of rules you should apply to sleeping if you are having trouble. Now, I've never had full-blown insomnia and I feel the utmost sympathy for any of you who deal with this regularly, but I was certainly up for fine-tuning the two- to three-hour blocks of sleep that I was getting each night. I did a little research on sleep hygiene and although it all seemed rather obvious I thought I should give it a go. I often find obvious advice is the most easily ignored, but it is often incredibly effective.

The rules seemed to all stem from one very simple one, which is that the bed should be exclusively the place for sleep and sex. No other activity should be thrown into the mix under that floral duvet! So out of the window goes breakfast in bed (although, to be honest, for me that went out of the window a long way before this set of rules came into my life. Two young kids will straighten that one out for you), binge-watching a box set on a Sunday evening or catching up on emails on a rainy day from the comfort of your mattress. For me, the biggest lump of bereavement came from the NO READING IN BED rule. That WAS my evening before I stumbled across this new theory. What the hell was I supposed to do in that commodious chunk of time that sat between dinner and sleep? I then realised I could read in the bath, which would be a second best to in bed and would have to do for now.

So rather than my bed being synonymous with stories, words and pondering after an hour reading my favourite novel, it would simply be a place relating to the big Zs. Could this simple mind game really work? It seems it has. I had about a week where I felt the urge to cheat in the same way you might want to quickly cram a large doughnut when you're supposed to be on a health kick. Would anyone find out if I read in bed? Would it really make a difference? Can I really be bothered with MORE rules?

I stuck to it, though, and as a result I only get up to go to the loo once a night on average. I still have moments where I know I haven't delved into a deep sleep but those nights occur much less often if I stick to this new sleep-hygiene mantra.

Going to bed at the right time was also a must, as we should be getting into the bed ready to fall straight to sleep. I was getting into bed way too early and then restimulating my mind before getting tired. It is apparently much better to keep your

CLEAR YOUR HEAD BEFORE BED

I don't always sleep so well so I find writing a list of everything that's in my head before I hit the hay very therapeutic. Write down in the space below everything that is filling up your mind. It could be tomorrow's shopping lists, people you need to call or bigger worries about the future. Get them out on to the paper and know you can deal with them after a good night's sleep.

....

....

....

....

....

....

....

....

body and mind working outside of the bedroom and to then head to bed when you really need it. The caveat to that is we should all try to keep high-energy activity down to a minimum in these pre-bed hours. So leaving a sizeable gap between sport and bed is a good idea if possible.

These days the most tempting cake on the plate is the smartphone! Just one more sneaky look at Instagram before bed. Just one more whizz through the online news before I shut off. All of these stimulating stories, ideas and photos are not giving our brains the right signals for a deluxe sleep. The light our phones give off is also a signal for the brain to be alert and think it's daytime, so there's another reason to shut down phones and laptops way before we plan to sleep. I actually set myself this rule a while ago; I like to keep on top of work emails so I would have my phone poised by my bedside, but I was so addicted to it I now turn off all devices at around 9p.m. and then turn my phone back on the next day. The world will not crumble if I don't reply to a work email or know what body part Kim Kardashian has flashed that day.

We are all too used to receiving all information all of the time and therefore our tolerance for others' delays in response is nil. We want answers and we want them quick. This kind of expectation can take us so far from calm. We have no patience or understanding of what else someone might be doing and we assume that others are being rude or lazy if the response doesn't arrive within the hour. Give yourself a break from the demands of your phone and let others off the hook, too. I'm still mastering this one but my goodness it helps with sleep.

SELF-CARE

Another key element to tap into calm is self-care. It is essential to our general wellbeing and we have to take responsibility for it, as no one else is going to do it for us.

Self-care to a Brit usually sends shivers up one's spine and makes our toes coil into the depths of our tightly tied shoes. Why are we culturally so bad at looking after ourselves? We see it as a luxury only prescribed to the elite or lucky, whereas it should be ingrained daily into all of our lives, no matter what we are going through. The usual excuses for lack of self-care in this day and age are . . .

I have no time.

I have too many others to care for.

I don't need to.

I'm far too busy for that . . .

We put self-care at the very bottom of the list of things to do each day, but how are we to get through all the things on the list to the best of our abilities if we aren't looking after ourselves? This is where so many of us trip up. We are so focused on others, the end goal or simply doing too much, that we lose sight of the obvious. What's the point of having a fab job if we are in ill-health because of it? What's the point of having a family that is well organised and educated if we can't enjoy life with them? What's the point of having a packed diary if we are too tired to enjoy it all?

We get so carried away with the 'must dos' and 'have tos' that we forget to get back to basics. I always find simplifying everything in life leads to calm. Some portions of our lives are quite simply unavoidably complex and intricate but there are other parts of our lives that we can change. We can ask for help, do a little less and recreate our own rule book.

If we know we are looking after ourselves to increase our optimum wellbeing, our bodies and minds are going to be much less stressed. If we are physically and mentally feeling good it is so much easier to act from a calm place, to make decisions wrapped in trust and to know that fundamentally we are okay. If we have pain, feel sick, are mentally exhausted or have hit a wall, everything else in life feels like a burden. Making small decisions can tip us over the edge, and the actions of others can make us want to hide away rather than calmly confront them, and life's speed can make us feel drained. Making sure we all give ourselves time and space to do what makes us feel good alleviates many other tricky areas in life and lets calm do its magic.

WHAT DOES SELF-CARE MEAN TO YOU?

Self-care is perhaps not as frivolous and luxurious an idea as you may assume. It doesn't have to involve going to a swanky spa for the day or rubbing expensive creams all over ourselves. To me, it is much simpler than that. The best way I can put it is to imagine myself as a friend. If a friend were to come to me telling me they were tired and drained I would tell them to rest up and take it easy. Sometimes if I feel depleted I won't let myself off the hook; I'll try to keep on pushing while my demons pop up to tell me I'm being lazy. Yet if I imagine a friend with the same complaint I know exactly what my advice would be.

If I'm feeling agitated and discombobulated I again try to imagine what I would tell a loved one. Perhaps I would suggest some fresh air and physical movement or an early night and a good comedy. We are so hard on ourselves, so imagining what we might tell someone else is a great way to get in touch with what we know deep down will work. It's all about being kind to ourselves, reducing how much we beat ourselves up about past mistakes and how we physically move and rest.

To me, self-care is about listening to our bodies so that we rest when they need rest, and get ourselves moving when our heads are spinning. It's about using simple tools to help get ourselves back on track, having made the decision from a loving place.

Self-care isn't overindulgent or a luxury, it's about not being too hard on yourself. I think in this day and age, especially for women, that can be tricky because there are numerous constant reminders as to what we could be achieving or feeling less guilty about. So many things we're supposed to be engaged with or striving for, so many things we feel we should be concerned with – anti-ageing, gaining muscle, losing weight, wearing the right clothes, climbing the ranks to the most powerful job, marrying the perfect partner, etc. The demands and pressures on ourselves are endless, therefore it is easy to slip into the world of compare and despair. Taking ourselves away from this constant churn of options allows us to just sit as we are and know that we are fine in the moment. We don't need to berate ourselves for being uneducated on a certain subject, not being able to tackle a problem head on, or for not having perfect hair. Always try to think about what advice you would give to someone you love, then apply it to yourself. That, right there, is self-care.

When I know I'm being too hard on myself I imagine what I would say to a friend and what advice I would give in a similar position. Below, write a letter to yourself imagining you are talking to a friend and see how much kinder, softer and forgiving you are. Then see if you can apply your advice and suggestions to the situation.

TO

SUBJECT

So how can we all ingrain this way of thinking into our everyday lives? First of all, try to wake up each morning with one positive thought about yourself. Start your day remembering one positive attribute or quirk that you cherish and celebrate it from the moment you open your eyes. If we start our day enjoying who we are, we set a precedent for the rest of the day. Listen to your body and see where you sit on your own barometer of wellbeing. If you are feeling boosted with energy and optimism, work to your best that day. Step out of your comfort zone knowing you've got the energy to do so. If you wake up feeling low in immunity, work to what your best is that day – it might be a lot lower than previous days but know that it's okay to not reach the heady heights today or to have to push yourself every day of the week. Allow yourself rest and recuperation when it is needed.

Lastly, go to bed knowing that you did your best. If mistakes were made, it doesn't matter, it's simply part of your story that's teaching you constantly. We can learn from mistakes, move on and try again. There are no exceptions to this on Earth. We all make mistakes and we all get the chance to try again. Don't beat yourself up, accept your actions and reactions and feel calm knowing you did your best.

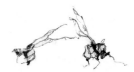

Summary

BE KIND TO YOURSELF.

Look after your body; fuel it properly and enjoy the way it moves.

SLEEP.

Don't see sleep as an optional extra, make time for it and acknowledge its power.

TUNE INTO YOUR BODY.

Take an inventory of every part of you and listen to what part needs care.

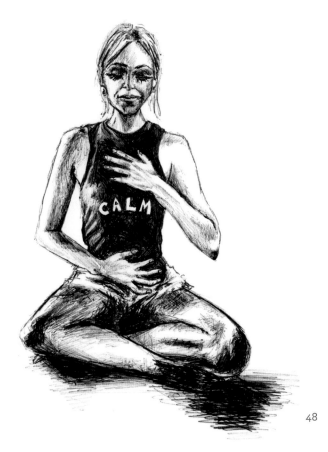

WHAT DOES A CALM BODY LOOK LIKE TO YOU?

Write one word or draw a picture here that sums it up.

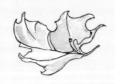

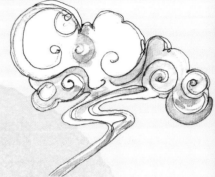

CALM
BREATH

Filling our lungs with air and letting it all out again is a reflex action and something we rarely give much thought or time to. So how hard can breathing be? How can you get it wrong? The resounding answers to these questions, when you dig a little deeper, are most definitely 'VERY' and 'In so many ways'! So many of us get into strange habits with how we let that vital air in and out of our bodies, myself included. Think back to the last time you were excited or stressed. It is very likely your breathing was either much quicker than normal or stopped in its tracks.

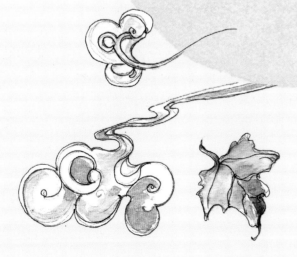

TYPES OF BREATHING

When I started writing this book, breathing was one of the areas I wanted to focus on. I touched on its importance in *HAPPY*, but after experiencing my panic attacks it was something I wanted to investigate in more depth, as the first thing I noticed during those few scary minutes was the notion of having no control over the short, sharp pants that were sending my whole body into panic. My lungs felt as if they were almost contracting rather than gently and calmly gathering the oxygen they needed. My instinct in these panic-saturated moments was to breathe deeper and more smoothly. I tried so hard to gulp down air into the pit of my stomach and to blow it out evenly but the panic that was controlling the show had other ideas and compressed my lungs further, ensuring only the smallest amount of air was allowed in and back out at any one time.

When I'm nervous I tend to do the exact opposite. If I'm faced with a colossal and nerve-wracking job and I'm delivering lines or about to speak, I tend to hold my breath at the top of my chest. The air sits there waiting for the impending moment of possible disaster and daren't leave my lungs in case that motion causes some problematic domino effect. If I stay as still as I can and hold my lungs and muscles tight then maybe I'll be steeled for what's to come and just maybe everything will go to plan. It's all very subconscious but since I started delving into this subject matter for the book, it's something I do that I'm much more aware of and intrigued by.

I've mentioned already the birthing technique I used during my second labour (with Honey). My friend Hollie de Cruz, a hypnobirthing expert, told me to imagine a large colourful balloon during my labour with Honey. She taught me that with each contraction I should breathe in and imagine the balloon expanding, and then taught me how to steadily release that breath. I'm not quite sure how the alchemy of this simple technique works but what I do know is that it was a game changer. It allowed me to calm my body and mind so that every inch of me believed everything was okay and that I would get through it. There were no mind tricks, nor was there a magical hippy-type waving a branch of sage over my face; I simply felt in control and calm because of my breathing. Yet even after this moment and learning how impactful conscious breathing could be, I somehow stored away that information in a corner of my mind reserved for 'childbirth', then carried on breathing in a very irregular fashion in my everyday life.

'LEARNING' TO BREATHE

So can someone teach you how to breathe? It turns out they really can! I discovered breathing coach Rebecca Dennis through a friend and intrigued and as research for this book, I went along to see her magic for myself. On page 58 you can find my interview with Rebecca and some of the breathing exercises she took me through, but briefly here, this is what I experienced:

Our minds are bulging with information, ideas, concerns, dreams and everything else in between. Sometimes it feels like a right old jumble sale in that brain. Write in the spaces in the pictures below what is on your mind and how your brain is feeling today.

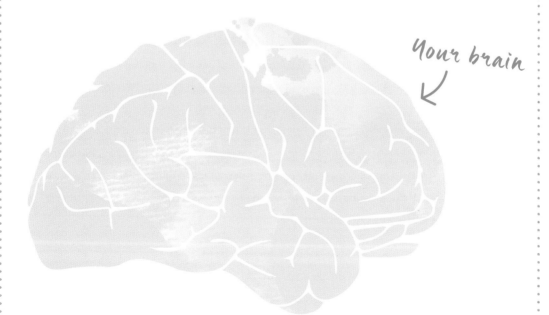

My brain →

A bit wired
Tired
Concerned
fidgety
Happy
Over stretched
Creative
A little Jumbled

Your brain ↙

When I arrived at the yoga studio where Rebecca works, I told the receptionist I had an appointment with her, which was met with a joyful smirk and slow nod. At this point I knew I was in for something special.

Rebecca talked me through her own incredible story and how she discovered the techniques that she now practises with many devotees. I was fascinated but still had not the foggiest as to what I was about to experience. She told me that by partaking in controlled and instructed breathing many inner emotions and past locked grievances, traumas or worries may be freed so that I could move on from them. She also told me to expect nothing and just let go and see what happens without too much thought.

I often wonder if this is our biggest problem in the modern world? We all THINK too much. It's constant: ideas, worries, concerns, comparisons, assumptions. It doesn't stop until we hit the sack, exhausted and all thought-out. Luckily I quite naturally switched off as soon as my session started with Rebecca, as I was so focused on getting the breathing technique right (TEACHER'S PET!) that all other thoughts stayed out on the busy London street where I'd left them. Time seemed meaningless during this whole escapade, so I can't be accurate as to when it all started to kick off, but soon after I got into this mystic cycle of breath everything seemed to open up. My chest lost its usual tightness, my windpipe seemed to expand and have more flow and my stomach softened and stopped trying to look flat and intact after childbirth. As Rebecca moved around my body on the floor, pressing specific pressure points and confirming strong mantras, I felt like a small alien under autopsy. I realised in this moment that I felt far from human in the way I had been carrying on. Pushing myself, never stopping, constantly thinking, invariably slightly stressed and disconnected.

Almost alien to the original state of what a human is. We all arrive on planet Earth untouched by experience, regret or trauma and are programmed to see joy, laughter and love, so how come so many of us travel so far from this place? As kids we roam, watch, listen, smell, seek joy always and have a need for fun in the moment. Rebecca was uncovering this and pushing out all of those modern stresses with her words and hands. I could feel it all dispersing and drifting away.

That was when the tears started to roll. Not dramatic, cinematic sobs, more like wild whimpers that ran out of me at great speed. Hot tears flowed as I felt the pain and stress of millions of moments pass through me. Flashes of childbirth, people who have caused me pain, worries that I harbour about people and places due to history, times I've felt crushed. It all came gushing out of these new open spaces.

PILE UP

I had several realisations while the floodgates were open. One was about just how easily small stressful moments pile up, meaning that when something tiny happens – maybe I get a parking ticket or feel a little tired – the stress is maximised and becomes slightly out of control. This is because those small moments sit like tiny canaries on the heads of gargantuan elephants of stress beneath. That mass is made up of many moments and feelings that have built up over time and have sat stagnant, until we realise that we really don't need them hanging around anymore. What an epiphany! I could let go of those small stresses that didn't serve me in any way. Those stresses that live in the past and have no steer or bearing on my life today.

Another realisation was that I don't like to admit to myself that I have been hurt. I feel very lucky that I have a roof over my head and food in my fridge and so far have my physical health, so why would I want to say aloud that I've been hurt? Could it really mean that much and do I really hold on to any of it anyway? I realised during the session that I definitely do and it makes up so much of the stress that I feel about life's banal, smaller problems.

I have been very hurt by certain individuals over the years. Some of these people may even still be in my life now, but this breathing session was making it clear that the pain I felt in certain circumstances was still leaching off my system and making everything else in life slightly greyer and spikier. I'm not looking for sympathy by admitting this to you, or even to myself – we've all been hurt by someone over the years – but what I realised was that it's okay to feel those emotions and say it aloud. The release verified those feelings for me and made me feel okay about acknowledging them.

But what I think I've also learned is that there's an expiry date for these emotions, and if we don't let go and learn to trust again we'll carry this big sack of shit around for far too long, unnecessarily. Recognising this pain and unleashing it from tiny pockets of my body felt liberating to say the least.

Towards the end of the session I felt lighter, more in touch with what was really going on with me and really tingly. I felt I could almost fly out of the room on a magic carpet of newfound space in my life.

The breathing exercises are quite obviously intensely powerful and are something I really want to keep up in my own time, but this session also allowed me to realise so much of what I was holding on to that was contributing to so much of the stress I was feeling every day. Letting go is the key, and that sometimes feels impossible, but I think awareness and a bit of self-love and patience could be the best starting place. I know there's a lot more I need to let go of and a whole heap of acceptance I need to grasp to truly put all this into action, but it feels exciting rather than daunting. My breathing adventures have only just begun.

This truly extraordinary mental and physical adventure has led me to ponder so many questions. On the next page, Rebecca explains her breathing magic and digs a little deeper on the subject.

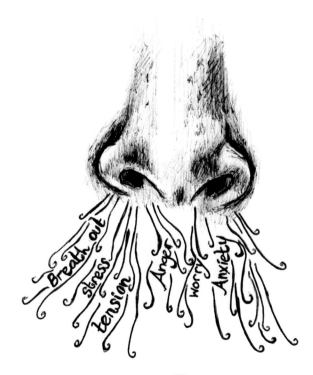

HELLO TO . . . REBECCA

F: Hello Rebecca, it has been so wonderful meeting you and experiencing your amazing Transformational Breath sessions. Can you tell us roughly what this sort of practice can offer up?

R: At the foundation of all breathing sessions is the practice of understanding our breathing patterns and deep breathing or 'belly breathing' – in which you allow your diaphragm to drop downwards and your rib cage to expand, creating more space for the lungs to inflate. In one of my sessions, I ask breathers to envisage breathing right down to their pelvic floors, starting with the breath expanding in the lower abdominals. Breathing in this way is also called 'deep diaphragmatic breathing', or 'conscious connected breathing', and it helps to balance the nervous system. When we activate our parasympathetic nervous system this is our calm state during which our heart rate slows, our blood pressure lowers and our blood supply is directed to nurture our digestive and reproductive systems rather than our muscles and brains. When our parasympathetic nervous system is active, our sympathetic nervous system – our 'fight or flight' state – becomes less active. This is the state that raises our heart rate, our blood pressure and respiratory rate to make us ready for action – and it is also responsible for releasing the stress hormones of adrenaline and cortisol into our bodies.

Many of us are unaware we are in fight or flight all the time or have feelings of low anxiety that we take for granted as a normal way of being. Human beings are designed to go into flight or fight if we are in danger or fleeing for our lives rather than when we open our email inbox or are under pressure with commitments. The problem is that most of us breathe in a rapid, short and shallow way all the time, or we are holding our breath regularly. A lot of clients I see are chest breathers and not breathing into their belly. This creates tension in the muscles that serve our respiratory system such as our shoulders, neck, throat and intercostals. We tend to guide our breath into our upper chest and no further, and fail to take advantage of our full lung capacity.

Founder of Transformational Breath and renowned breath expert, Dr Judith Kravitz, who has studied the way people breathe for the past 40 years agrees and says that in her experience most people are only using about 25–30 per cent of their lung capacity.

Breathing is something we all know how to do, and yet the majority of teenagers and adults let go of their natural ability to breathe fully. We are conditioned from an early age to control our feelings and emotions, and as a result our muscles tighten and our breathing patterns become restricted. The impact on our mental and physical wellbeing is huge.

By learning to consciously connect to our breath and encourage its natural rhythms, we can harmonise the body and mind, live life fully, find emotional freedom and feel calm and centred. Breathing can heal on many levels and of course our breath is constantly life-sustaining – taking in oxygen, invigorating red blood cells and expelling carbon dioxide, which is a metabolic waste product.

The first thing we do when we make our entrance into the world is breathe, and it is the last thing we do when we exit, so we may as well have a good relationship with the way we do this. We are all unique and we all have our own breathing pattern, a bit like our thumb print. Our breath pattern shows how we function in the world and what our coping mechanisms are. As a breath coach I am trained to read those patterns.

Babies are perfect breath gurus, and observing them means observing what an open healthy breath should be. Babies are so present, they don't have the 50,000 thoughts a day that we do as adults, and when you see them lying in a cot you will notice their breath is in their belly, midsection and chest and there are no blockages or restrictions. The same is true of toddlers, however, the majority of teenagers and adults are either chest breathers, belly breathers, shallow breathers or breath holders. Research shows that we only use around 33 per cent of our respiratory system. Conscious connected breathing helps us to understand and clear these restricted breathing patterns. By practising this technique we open up our respiratory system to its full capacity and this helps our overall wellbeing on a physical, mental and emotional level.

F: How can an awareness around our breathing help us in life?

R: Breathwork is much like therapy but without having to do the talking, which for some is a welcome relief. It's not about going over and over the story, but letting it go. Our experiences are our perception, and with this work we are accessing the conscious and subconscious mind. Our body is like a biological recording of our past and when we experience emotions such as fear or anger or feeling stressed, for example, our physiology can go into chaos. Our heart rate increases, our muscles tense, our digestion and immune system may be affected. We activate our sympathetic nervous system, our fight or flight mechanism, and release adrenaline and cortisol. Our body remembers everything and holds on to these memories. Think of when your body freezes or reacts and you feel triggered by events or people in certain situations. Data is constantly streamed down to the body from the brain and vice versa and is stored like a computer.

Just as we blink our eyes, our heart beats and our digestive system works, we breathe automatically. When we become aware of our breath we can control and be conscious of how we breathe. That can be really empowering and helps us to feel calm, centred and relaxed.

F: How did you stumble across this game-changing practice and how has it enhanced your own life?

R: I lived with depression for over 20 years, 15 of which were spent on prescribed medication. I reached a point in my 30s where I had tried and failed with so many therapies from CBT, psychotherapy to yoga and other alternative ways, I knew I needed help but I didn't know how to get it.

The black dog of depression jumped on my back when I was in my teens. Back in the 1980s, depression was taboo and people chose not to discuss it as there was a real stigma attached. I used to watch people going about their everyday life and quietly wonder if they felt as bad as I did. At my lowest point, I would go to a very dark place and feel that life was no longer worth living. On those days, I was just existing, watching the clock and wishing the day away. I had no sense of living in a healthy, vital way. I would on occasion have suicidal thoughts. Unable to share these irrational thoughts (like many depressed people, I didn't want to burden others), I would hide away, avoiding contact, feeling numb, disconnected and in despair at not being able to shift the mood. You can't show people you are feeling unwell if you are depressed. You don't have a plaster cast or a bandage.

Two months before I discovered Transformational Breath, I attempted to take my own life with a combination of pills and alcohol and ended up in hospital. Thankfully, it wasn't my time.

The first time I walked into a breath workshop, I didn't know what to expect. I'll try to describe my first experience. I could feel every cell in my body releasing and letting go. Physically, mentally and emotionally, I was in a complete state of flux. I was crying and sweating and my whole body was reverberating and vibrating. It was intense! I had no control and totally surrendered to the maelstrom of emotions and physical reactions.

Afterwards, I felt lighter and, for the first time in a very long time, I was full of hope. I also noticed I could make decisions more clearly and felt really positive. Realising I had been introduced to something very special I wasn't going to let it disappear from my life.

I want to stress that none of this happened overnight. I used the breath technique I had been taught every day and worked closely with my doctor. Medication was simply not working for me but for others it is necessary and you should always be guided by a doctor. Sometimes I'd have dark episodes and wonder if I should go back on medication, but I never did.

I began to feel whole, complete and physically present. My mind was clearer and my emotions were more balanced. Breathwork gave me my life back. It helped me to enhance other practices by being more present during yoga and letting go of my often destructive mind during meditation. After years of suffering with anxiety and chronic depression I discovered the healing power of my breath. My experiences have furnished me with an understanding and empathy for others, and my daily reward is my continuing journey and observing life-changing transformations with my clients by using breathwork.

F: How much do you think we underestimate the power of breath?

R: We totally underestimate our breath. I am always blown away by how powerful it is. We can heal ourselves on many levels simply by connecting to our breath. I have witnessed too many beautiful moments to mention where people have finally let go of physical and emotional pain, and the magic that comes with that can often be a deep and profound spiritual connection to whatever that person finds. We are all on some level seeking inner peace, and this to me is a fast-track way to getting there. We all have different belief systems – be it religion, connection to the divine, a god, the universe, self or nature – and our breath can help us to deepen that connection. Good breathing helps us feel more confident and able to let go of old belief systems and negative thought patterns that no longer serve us. Releasing old stories and past dramas previously held on to on a subconscious level gives us emotional depth. As if that isn't enough, breath can also reinvigorate sexual energy, deepen creative expression, improve sleep patterns and lower blood pressure.

The quality of our breath helps to relax the mind and enhance the ability to learn, focus, concentrate and memorise. The brain requires a great deal of oxygen to function and breathwork helps us to achieve clarity, feel grounded and be productive. It also relieves stress, anxiety, depression and negative thought patterns. Breathing properly can help us overcome addictive patterns of behaviour and eating disorders as well as igniting creativity and passion.

A statistic for you: we inhale and exhale around 20,000 times a day, yet most of us pay little attention to how we breathe or how deeply it affects us. In our increasingly demanding and complex world very few people are aware of the detrimental effects that improper breathing can have on our health and general wellbeing.

To balance work commitments, lifestyle and family life can be challenging. There is a lot of pressure in today's society for everyone to perform, and there seems to be just one pace of life – fast. In modern-day life we are tied to our phones, our laptops, our iPads. In a world where we are more connected than ever with people through the internet and social media, people feel more alone and disconnected.

The pattern goes a bit like this: life happens, we are multitasking, hitting deadlines, and certain situations put us under pressure. As a result, we are burning more energy than we need to, just taking care of business. Stimulation, activity and demands are all around us. We are on high-speed-runaway-train mode and our responsibilities, commitments and worries prevent us feeling calm and staying in the moment.

Sometimes we literally forget to take a breath. We find ourselves thinking, 'I'm so stressed out, I can't breathe', or we feel a tightness in our chest and feel 'I just need some space to breathe'. This is where conscious breathing comes in as an effective method of reducing stress.

How we breathe is indicative of how we feel about life. Our breath patterns correlate to every emotion, thought and experience. Think about when we are happy and relaxed, the breath feels free and easy. When we are feeling sad or depressed, however, our breath is shallow. When we are angry or fearful our breath pattern also changes and our body's chemistry reacts and takes action.

These breathing techniques are like taking the breath to the gym or for an MOT. We need to take care of our body in the way we do a vehicle in order for it to run smoothly, and in that way we are resetting and recalibrating the systems of our mind and body with the breath.

F: In my sessions with you I have felt a huge sense of release as energy and emotion pours out. How exactly does this technique work?

R: Breathwork is about feeling everything rather than analysing and overthinking it, and often that can be uncomfortable – but releasing and cathartic, too. Emotion is simply energy in motion. Often we suppress and repress our emotions and we hold onto them or we push them down until they come up again. Heavier emotions, such as grief or anger, can disrupt our lives when they stay with us. For example, we hold on to repressed emotions in our jaw and some people may grind their teeth at night. Others feel emotion in the belly, such as fear or butterflies, which can affect our digestive system and cause issues such as IBS. We carry a lot of tension in our shoulders and our body which can play havoc with the mind. Our body has an innate intelligence and is constantly sending messages to let us know when something is happening, although often we miss the signs.

Thoughts can be just as toxic as some of the things we consume and the breath helps us to release these toxins through our exhale. When we are connecting to our breath we are creating a circuit that can access that lower, denser energy and raise the vibrations so we can integrate them.

F: How can we all use breath in everyday life to improve our general wellbeing?

R: The more we notice the rhythm of our inhale and exhale the more we understand our patterns. Just being aware of our breath can be helpful in everyday life, when we are at home, walking outside, watching TV, cooking, on our commute, in the bath or at the office. Ideally creating a practice every day can make a real difference, even if it's just for one to two minutes each day. (If we put pressure on ourselves to have a daily one-hour meditation practice it may feel like a chore or not realistic and we give up before we have even begun!) We can make things simple by walking and using that time to meditate with each step, just by being aware of our breath. I find that running, using different breathing exercises and swimming is my meditation. There are no rules and it's about finding what works best for you.

F: When we feel stressed or anxious the first thing that seems to alter is our breathing. How do we get more conscious and back on track with our breathing and how will this stabilise us?

R: Stress can be positive, keeping us alert and ready to avoid danger. It helps us to get the job done and only becomes negative when we face continuous challenges without relief or relaxation in between. As a result, we become overworked and stress-related tension starts to build.

Often when we feel stressed or anxious our breathing speeds up and we breathe more into our chest area. We may feel different sensations in our body or we start to feel a little hot or flustered. Try to become the observer of your feelings and notice where your breath is. Take some deep diaphragmatic breaths into the belly. Inhale through the nose and out of the mouth with a little pause in between. As you breathe in, expand your belly and as you exhale the belly goes in. This will help you to be more focused and centred and bring you back into the moment. *"*

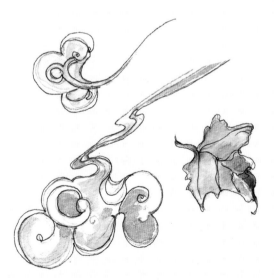

SOME BREATHING EXERCISES
BY REBECCA DENNIS

1) TO RELAX AND CALM THE MIND

- Sit or lie down in a comfortable, quiet spot where you won't be disturbed.

- Close your eyes and ensure your shoulders and jaw are relaxed and the spine is straight.

- Take a long deep exhalation out of your mouth.

- Close your mouth and inhale deeply through your nose, directing the breath deep into the belly – visualise filling a balloon of air in your centre as you do this.

- Exhale gently through the mouth – visualise the balloon gently deflating as you do this.

- Notice any sensations that arise in the body – acknowledge them and gently bring your attention back to your breath.

- Be aware of your thoughts, and rather than trying to push them away, gently push them aside and come back to the inhale and exhale.

- Visualise the breath calming and relaxing the mind and all the systems of the body, and as you exhale allow it to release any tension.

- Try to do this for 15 minutes, and notice the difference it makes to your day.

2) ANXIOUS ALARM CALL

Woken up early again? It's 4a.m. and you are wide awake with lists going through your head and you can't get back to sleep. Try this simple but effective exercise to regain a sense of calm. It really works.

Breathe in through your nose for four seconds, hold your breath for seven seconds, then exhale through your mouth for eight seconds. This helps us to come out of the mind, slow the heart rate and activate the parasympathetic nervous system to bring us into a relaxed state.

3) A BREATHING EXERCISE FOR THOSE OF YOU WITH EMAIL OVERLOAD

You open your inbox and there are 100 emails waiting for you. Where to begin? Try this exercise to centre and balance your mind.

Close your eyes. Place your thumb over your right nostril and exhale through the left nostril for eight counts. Breathe in through the left nostril and hold for another eight. Now repeat on the other side. Keep going up to 10 times and notice the difference in your breath.

4) AN EXERCISE FOR CREATING SPACE IN THE MIND

'By letting it go it all gets done. The world is won by those who let it go. But when you try and try the world is beyond winning.' Lao Tzu

Often we spend a lot of time in our thoughts and sometimes experience recurring negative thought patterns. Don't believe everything your mind is telling you, sometimes it is very destructive. Here's a very simple exercise to help you let go of the mind clutter so that you can create room for clarity and calm.

First, leave all your thoughts at the door. Whatever it is you have to do today or tomorrow or should have done and perhaps haven't managed to yet, leave it all at the door. You can return to this later.

- Close your eyes and sit up straight.

- Feel the ground beneath your feet and your sitting bones on the seat beneath you.

- Relax your shoulders and let out a deep sigh.

- Begin to notice the breath and become aware of the inhale and the exhale.

- Imagine the breath is coming in and out like a wave.

- Breathe softly and deeply in through the nose and out through the nose with a little pause in between.

- As you inhale, guide the breath into the belly, encouraging a deep diaphragmatic breath.

- Allow the mind to wander to the breath and each time you notice you're going back into thoughts, take the mind back to the breath.

- Begin to draw your focus and attention to the rise and fall of your breath.

- Allow the breath to flow – you are not forcing it or pushing it. Gentle breathing.

- Expand your awareness inside and let go of the outside.

- There is nowhere to go, nothing to do, just stay present with your breath.

- Everything is as it should be right now, there is no wrong and there is no right.

- Stay present with your inhale and your exhale.

- Notice any thoughts that are there and gently push them aside.

- Step outside of the thoughts and observe them.

- Do not entertain them, just allow them to pass like clouds in the sky.

- Breathe in and breathe out, letting go of anything that no longer serves you.

- Exhale away any tension or worries.

- Inhale in new energy, positivity and light.

- Let go of the pull of the future and the pull of the past.

- Continue to go deeper inside, explore and expand your awareness inside with each breath.

- Stay in this moment, which is NOW.

- Keep practising this for two to three minutes, then notice how your mind feels.

Summary

TAKE A BREAK.

CHUCK OUT EMOTIONAL BAGGAGE.

. . . AND BREATHE!

Notice your own breathing patterns and how they change when you're stressed.

Don't be trapped by your emotions – let it out, then let it go.

Give one of Rebecca's exercises a go when you're feeling stressed.

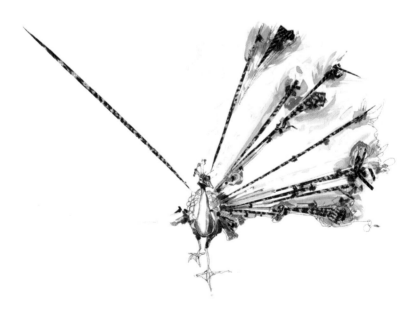

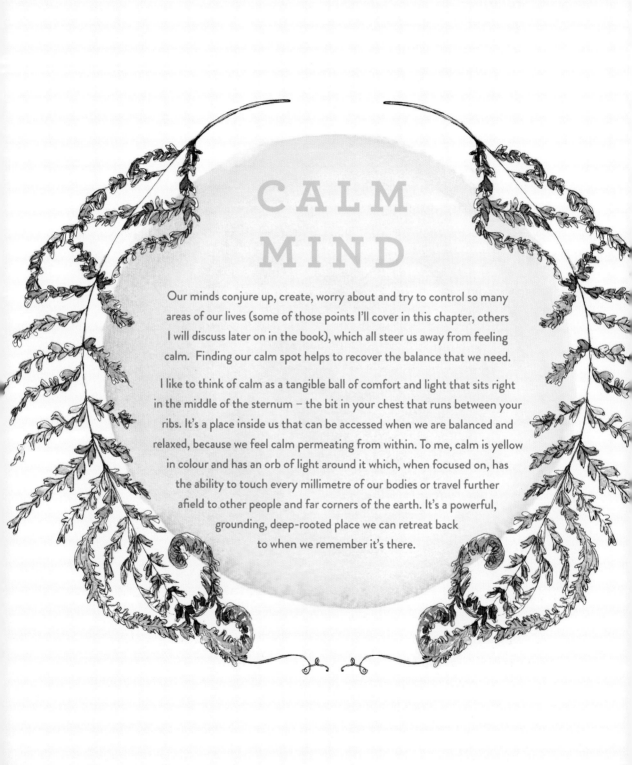

CALM MIND

Our minds conjure up, create, worry about and try to control so many areas of our lives (some of those points I'll cover in this chapter, others I will discuss later on in the book), which all steer us away from feeling calm. Finding our calm spot helps to recover the balance that we need.

I like to think of calm as a tangible ball of comfort and light that sits right in the middle of the sternum – the bit in your chest that runs between your ribs. It's a place inside us that can be accessed when we are balanced and relaxed, because we feel calm permeating from within. To me, calm is yellow in colour and has an orb of light around it which, when focused on, has the ability to touch every millimetre of our bodies or travel further afield to other people and far corners of the earth. It's a powerful, grounding, deep-rooted place we can retreat back to when we remember it's there.

LOCATING THE SWEET SPOT

Why do we forget this spot is there? The distraction of life. We are constantly taken away from this sweet spot because there seems to be so much going on around us. Chores to be done, appointments to be made, people to see, work to be finished, people to look after, social media to gobble up, things to buy, goals, dreams, desires, wants. DISTRACTIONS. All of these things we think we need to focus on constantly take us away from calm. What's this got to do with the mind? Well, I like to think that geographically the brain is not far from calm at all – it would sit just over a ruler's length away from this delicious spot in our bodies. Yet the brain has the habit of taking us far, far away from this place to the point of feeling as if we might not be able to access it ever again. My mind is at times capable of flinging me intergalactic distances, to a place where I feel unrooted, chaotic and far away from home. That calm space within us IS home, yet our minds can catapult us in the exact opposite direction in seconds.

If things at home feel chaotic and I am chasing my tail with the kids and my career and I know I'm not giving enough time to my marriage or friendships, I feel myself moving away from that sweet spot within. My feet hover above the ground and I scramble to make sense of all the intricate parts of life that make up my world. My mind throws around ideas and worries which make me travel further and further away from home. Those little voices telling me I'm not good enough and that I'm failing in areas of my life. Thoughts of past mistakes mean I quickly descend into feelings of panic and fear. We may try to battle these thoughts and feelings, but then the ego pipes up and gives us even more reason to not listen to our instinct and our calm within.

The ego – not the 'big-headed' ego, but the 'low-self-esteem' ego – loves moments like this. It's his perfect moment to shout about all of the self-centred concerns that don't really matter. The ego will grab hold of these weak spots and wring out any self-love or confidence as he knows you're perhaps not strong enough to cancel out his words. The ego works purely from shallow depths and only cares for the superficial in life. The coal for his fire are all of your self-doubts and concerns, which he'll whip into a frenzied fire that rages on until we route back to calm. Ego can't breathe in calm, so he has no choice but to retreat back to his darkened shallows. Some might assume ego is all about boasting and arrogance, but it is so much more complex than that. Even if the ego is illuminating bravado and confidence, it's nearly always coming from a place of lacking and fear. Proper confidence comes from love, not fear, so there's the BIG difference.

CHOOSING THE RIGHT ROUTE

So, in these moments, how do we turn the compass and navigate back to that place of grounded ease? First up, you need to know that you can. There are no exceptions. It'll take some of us longer to do this than others – it might be harder for some to let go of habitual negative patterns – but we can all get there if we really want to. Some of us love the drama of a calm-less mental space because it feels comfortable and worn in. It might be what you are used to, so it feels like a huge wrench to leave it behind. It's a personal decision to see life in a new way and to try new ways of thinking, just remember it is YOUR choice. And if you're ready, go for it.

There are many options to choose from if you are up for routing back to calm, but some are more short-lived than others, with no guarantees of where we will travel to afterwards. If we feel stressed and choose, say, a bottle of wine to quell the frantic thoughts and worries, we are likely to drop from the heightened state of stress but it may not have lasting results. The alcohol will wear off and we will end up where we started, but perhaps with a hangover to boot! We all know our own weaknesses and how we attempt to combat them, and it'll be different for each of us, so we have to try to swerve past these urges when we feel particularly far from calm and look for new routes; the pathways which will lead us directly back to that warm ball of light and feeling of being grounded, but in a longer-lasting, gentle manner.

SURVIVING TRAUMA

Something I also really wanted to talk about in this book is the effects of trauma and how it can drown out calm. When trauma strikes it is often shocking, overwhelming and unfortunately has lasting effects. I'm not talking about missing a flight or scratching the side of the car on a wall, I'm talking about life-altering episodes that leave bruises way under the surface of the skin. Trauma can arrive in so many forms but the mental scars that are left behind are usually pretty similar.

I've had to surface after trauma in my own life. Time has helped me to heal and get back on my feet so that I could walk away from pain, stress and upset. Weeks and months rhythmically moving me on and the support of great friends and family

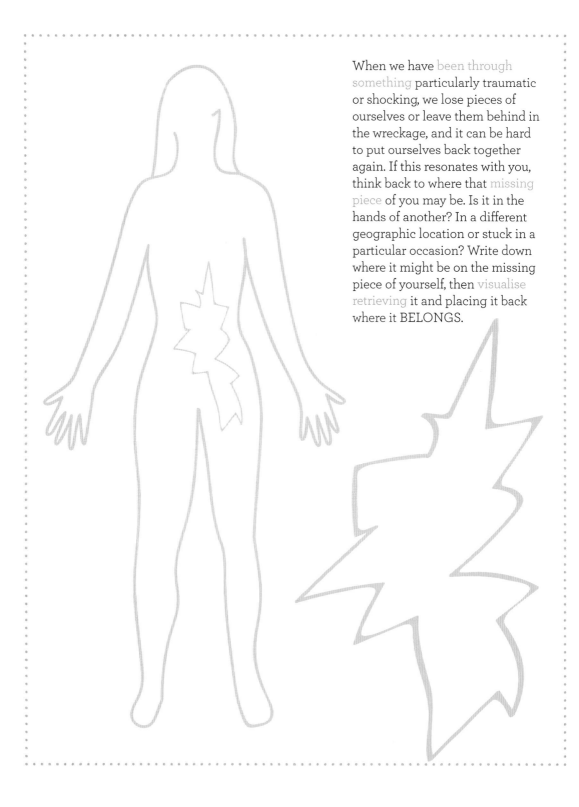

When we have been through something particularly traumatic or shocking, we lose pieces of ourselves or leave them behind in the wreckage, and it can be hard to put ourselves back together again. If this resonates with you, think back to where that missing piece of you may be. Is it in the hands of another? In a different geographic location or stuck in a particular occasion? Write down where it might be on the missing piece of yourself, then visualise retrieving it and placing it back where it BELONGS.

members helped a lot, but not completely. When you've experienced trauma there are still haunting moments or instant reminders that drag you back to the source of your pain and suffering in a nanosecond. If you've had a bad car accident with a yellow mini, for example, you might shudder every time you see that type of car. If you've lost a loved one out of the blue, the mention of their name or smell of their perfume may fling you back to the moment of loss all over again. Although we can move on and live in the now, there is an element of brain muscle memory which might still need work so that you are able to let go that little bit more.

I have a lovely friend named Yvonne Williams, a counsellor who deals with many clients who have post-traumatic stress disorder (PTSD). During one enlightening conversation Yvonne likened trauma to a shattering glass. Our bodies and souls smash into tiny fragments when we go through such a situation, and our work then is to put ourselves back together. We may do a good job of building ourselves back up, but there could be a tiny fragment of us still lying on the floor where the trauma took place.

Yvonne asked me to visualise where this tiny fragment of me could be. I instantly pictured it and felt sad. She asked me to visualise heading to the scene to pick it up. The experience was truly emotional: I saw myself walking over to this small part of myself and collecting it like a lonely child waiting at the school gates. I held that part of me close and will continue to because it calms me down massively and is helping me to heal properly. If I'm having a tough time or feel the stresses of my past catching up with me, I now know where to look for that missing piece and how to get back on my feet. This simple visualisation is a very powerful tool if you have been through anything traumatic.

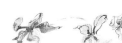

HELLO TO . . . YVONNE

Y: PTSD is recollections of stressful events or traumas. It's a complex disorder which affects a person in different, various ways. There are so many different circumstances which can bring this disorder into being, and it's never an identical process. Some may have a few symptoms, others a whole and varied set of distressing reactions. It is, however, manageable and a great deal of sensitive and skilled healing applications can truly help enormously.

F: What are the symptoms of PTSD?

Y:The symptoms of PTSD present in various ways. You may re-experience the traumatic event, have flashbacks and nightmares, but huge emotional shifts (anger, fear, irritability), tears, physical inbalance, muscle aches and physical weakness are not uncommon.

On a physical level the nervous system is deeply affected – people move into 'fight or flight' mode. The fear can actually immobilise them, and there is sometimes a regression into the 'inner child' self - feeling absolutely helpless and scared and out of control. The brain races to find a solution, so the patterns of thought can become muddled, disturbed and confusing and this of course can heighten the sense of trauma, and there is the potential to get 'stuck' in the experience again.

F: Other than physically, how else can it affect us?

Something I call 'soul loss' can occur. The fragmentation of the soul – or whatever you like to call your inner conscience. The individual can feel very lost following the trauma. Skilled professionals and healers can assist with the recovery of this fragmentation, so that those who feel they have 'jumped out' out of their body can come back to it through sensitive healing, such as vibrations and positive energy.

F: How much of PTSD is about cognitive recall?

Y: The mind is a powerful tool and memories of trauma can be triggered by any one of the senses. The thought process can be helped and healed to realign itself with CBT (Cognitive Behavioural Therapy). This is one of the most powerful tools, but there are others as well – sourcing appropriate help can actually also help and heal in itself as it becomes part of the re-empowering process.

F: How can a person get help in healing and recovering from trauma and its lasting effects?

Y: The help available for PTSD is vast – specifically trained trauma therapists can be sourced and they will be able to expertly work with their client in a safe space that allows understanding and healing. Mediation, yoga, soul retrieval, breathwork, relaxation techniques, nature and music also are very powerful for the soul and mind.

Guided visualisations can also be an effective experience if you are that way inclined, otherwise music, art therapy and creativity can be equally effective. In terms of music, I have found the solfeggio frequencies with their specific vibrations are very good for soothing and healing.

F: What would you say to someone who thinks they may have PTSD but isn't sure?

Y: PTSD presents in many different circumstances and the awareness of this now is more prevalent, which means there is lots of compassionate understanding for those seeking help and healing. Don't be afraid to ask for it.

THE IMAGINATION
ROAD TRIP

Visualisations can be so very helpful in healing and moving on in life. I have a vivid imagination which paints pictures of future plans and ideas with thick, definite brush strokes and luminous colour. Saying that, this passionate part of my mind also has the capability to act like that friend you had at college who was a bit of a liability. That friend who would embellish, exaggerate and lead you off your path and into trouble. This is another unruly part of my head that I find tricky to tame because I don't want to dilute its energy or importance as I use that part of it to dream and create. I just need to try to stop it running away wildly from grounded, positive calm thoughts.

I'll give you an example of one of my imagination's road trips. Every now and then my husband will be away for work so I'll find myself climbing into bed, with my children snoring nearby, feeling pretty exhausted and ready for a night of rest. All of a sudden my imagination will start to creak into gear and I'll receive flashes of pictures of every window in the house fully open. Now I know every window is shut but now my imagination is playing tricks with my memory and making me second-think my previous actions. Out of bed I get to go and check all windows are firmly locked. Then I'll slip back into bed only for my imagination to remind me of the oven and all that I've cooked that day. I clearly remember turning off all the knobs on the hob but now my imagination has grabbed hold of panic and is blurring my memories of how and when I last cooked. I'd better go check. This goes on for some time and I usually end up going to bed feeling slightly wired and unsettled. The only thing that will soothe me in these moments is visualisation. I imagine a giant angel with huge, white, feathered wings perched on top of the roof of our house. Its wings drape down over the sides of the house and its soft, calm smiles stares down at us all sleeping below. If I really focus on this image my imagination softens and stops running away with itself and I can eventually get some sleep.

Other times my imagination will convince the more grounded parts of my brain that I'm seriously ill. I'll panic that I've got a deadly disease that will see me finished off by the end of the year. I will feel breathless and physically exhausted from this blast of imagination which is not particularly conducive to staying healthy in the first place. I again try to visualise white light coming out of my body and warmth all around the surface of my skin. I try to bring my thoughts back to gratitude and physical comfort until my imagination quietens down and stops the sheer panic.

Visualisation can be very helpful in these moments of mental chaos and help bring us quite quickly back to calm. Sometimes panic can feel very detached, as if you have left your physical body altogether. Getting rooted back to your physical self and feeling grounded is so important in these moments. It sounds almost too simple but it works for me. If you ever feel panicky, anxious or stressed, give it a go. And if these particular visualisations don't work for you, pick your own narrative. It could be imagining a still pond of water inside you that flattens out like a sheet of glass, never moving and deep within you, or it could be imagining a hand gently pushing your shoulders down away from your ears and holding you calm and still. Whatever it is, picture it vividly and believe in its power.

CHANNEL THE POWER
OF YOUR MIND

Whilst we're on the subject of our powerful minds, have you ever been in a situation where something really needed to happen? Perhaps you were late for work and you could see your bus readying to leave the bus stop, your last-chance saloon to make it to the office on time. Somewhere deep inside your mind a voice said 'YOU CAN GET THAT BUS, GO! RUN LIKE USAIN BOLT AND MAKE THAT BUS' and you did make it, in fact quite easily.

Maybe you needed to pick up something terribly heavy and were on your own. Your mind gave you that belief you could do it and you somehow gained that extra bit of strength.

Maybe you have run a marathon and at the 23-mile point felt your tender legs giving way beneath you. Your mind may have stepped in and said 'COME ON! WE CAN DO THIS! NOT FAR NOW' which powered you on for the last three gruelling miles.

For me, that situation was writing a book. I wasn't sure that I could do it or that anyone would read it but my mind kept telling me softly, 'you can do this, just keep writing. Don't feel judged at this point, just write, write, write.' So I did. My mind gave me permission to calm those negative thoughts and I was able to override the devil on my shoulder. Those negative voices cause unnecessary stress because they only speak of what MIGHT happen, not what is actually happening. If we dig deep we can find our inner confidence and work with a calm, realistic mind. I'm so glad I listened to my gut and not my mind back then because the result was *HAPPY*, a book which was a joy to write for me, and I hear from so many of you that it brings you happiness too.

So get that mind on board and reach for those words that encourage and cheer-lead you all the way. Ignore the negative thoughts and 'what if's and listen to the positive words that come from your place of inner calm! Know the difference and you're onto a winner.

LET IT GO

There are some other pertinent words that we can focus on and remember. They are – for some of us – such difficult words to really put into action and are sometimes annoying to hear from others: 'let go.'

At times I feel so uptight and I worry that if I stop thinking and planning my world will fall apart. What if I forget that one thing I need to make my day run smoothly? What if I'm not brainstorming my next project and keeping my brain active? What if I don't learn anything new today? What if I stopped vehemently disliking that person who makes me feel uncomfortable? What would really happen if I simply stopped? God, it can be relentless upstairs in that brain! This is when we can again descend into a whirlwind of chaos and worry rather than flow through our days.

How do we get that balance between being methodical and engaged yet still be able to stop to enjoy what is going on around us? I know I can get very bogged down with house chores, millions of scrawly lists I've made on scraps of paper, schedules for the kids and plans for us as a family. I cram so much into my head that I forget to actually enjoy it as it all pans out. I like to be organised (I blame that on being a Virgo or my incredibly together mother) so this sometimes takes paramount position over simply LIVING. Usually this sort of behaviour winds up in me getting irate because something didn't go to plan, and this can spur on a small tantrum like a petulant child, which definitely doesn't get me anywhere close to that grounded calm place. I know all this yet I still find myself getting wound up into the same state of stress and disarray.

It's times like this when I most definitely need to let go. Life will create obstacles, life will throw the unexpected at us and life will not listen to our lists and plans. Sure, write those lists and create those personal maps, but be prepared to veer away from them when life gives us the opportunity to do so. When we go off on a tangent, this is when our mind needs to be flexible, open and up for change. We'll talk more about change in the 'unexpected' chapter towards the end of the book.

Letting go can feel completely unnatural and massively destabilising, especially if, like me, you feel hectic and a little panicked when you're not in control. This is where you have to reinforce your new carefree state with TRUST! If we can completely trust in life and whatever it throws at us we can let go. This doesn't mean believing and expecting everything to be perfect, but trusting that we will learn from and accept whatever situations may arise. Control makes us believe there will be a certain outcome, which often leads to disappointment and sorrow when that is not the case. Although I know the rules I'm desperately trying to grasp this concept. Trust is the key! That's the ticket back to calm!

EXPERIMENTING WITH MEDITATION

One very obvious way of calming that frenetic old brain is mediation. I dip in and out of using this widely practised method and constantly promise myself THIS WILL BE THE YEAR I MEDITATE MORE. If you think meditation isn't your thing, give it a go. Meditating doesn't have to be about sitting on the floor crosslegged trying to make your mind go blank, the idea is simply to find some calm and get your brain to quieten down. I sometimes repeat a mantra in my head while I'm meditating so that I have one simple focus, which helps me clear all the other thoughts whirling around my mind. My mantra might go something like this: 'I AM GOOD ENOUGH. I AM ENOUGH.'

Focusing on these words gives me a chance to escape the firework display of thoughts popping out of the top of my head and some much-needed respite in this crazy world that we live in, even if it's just five minutes before bed. I'll repeat it over and over for a few minutes until every inch of me believes it, and then I drop off to sleep. I also often listen to guided meditations online. There are many to choose from so if I'm feeling groggy and know I'm working into the evening that day I might type into the search engine, 'meditation for rest'. Or if I'm run down and feeling the physical yelp of fatigue, I might type in, 'meditation for healing'. Then I tune in, concentrate on the words and let my mind focus on them. All other thoughts, worries and concerns make way for positivity and calm.

The other form of meditation is to try to banish all thoughts for an extended period of time. I find this so tough as my mind is like a feral dog wanting to break any rules enforced. This is one of the reasons why I REALLY need to give more time to meditation; it most definitely becomes easier to slip into and much more natural the more you do it. Meditation sessions, even when irregular, can work as a little spa day for the mind. A chance to stop, recharge and gain space and clarity. I sometimes bargain with my own mind and remind it that if it complies accordingly for the next ten odd minutes and clears out then perhaps it will be treated with a new exciting idea or sense of clarity it hasn't experienced before. Again, like a small puppy, my brain needs that incentive and structure.

If you've never given it a try and think it could lead you back to a calmer place, do short spells of meditation to start with. Go to your favourite room in your home and lower the lights or turn them off and light a candle. Making the room as cosy, comfy and atmospheric as you can always helps to set the scene. Sit comfortably in a chair with all your limbs relaxed and not touching anyone else. I prefer to lie down, much like at the end of a yoga class, on a mat or on my bed, with my back flat and my arms at my side. Once you're comfortable you just need to close your eyes, relax and slow your breathing, then let each thought slip away. At first thoughts will roll in like crashing waves. 'EEEK, I haven't hung the washing out... Maybe I'll wear my new trousers tomorrow ... Shall I cook tonight or get a takeaway?' Just let these thoughts roll in, then let them fade away as quickly as they came. Perhaps picture them floating off in bubbles – they can come back to you at a more convenient time that way.

This is a good way to start getting in to the swing of meditation even if you spend the whole 10 minutes or so just batting off thoughts. This technique becomes slicker and quicker the more you do it, so when those thoughts appear they recede to leave bigger, wider gaps of nothingness. You can also visualise something that resonates with you. I often see a large eye in between where my eyes rest when shut. I focus on this eye and let the colours change and the shapes morph. The more I zone in on this visual, the fewer thoughts come busting through the door. Just do what feels right for you, it's not a competition or a race to master the technique, even if you just manage a few minutes here and there, it's a jolly good start. You may feel fidgety or bored when you first give it a go, but that is just the mind trying to tell you that this is an unnecessary hobby. It doesn't like to be silenced so it will try with all its might to distract and disarm you and your calm efforts. In these moments remember how much all the other parts of your body are screaming out for this quiet; they just don't have the voice to articulate it quite so eloquently. The mind and its chatter will talk over the silence but the more you do it, the more the mind gets on board with meditation and realises it needs that break.

Give it a whirl and see what works for you, then reap the benefits of a clear and calmer mind.

Meditating can feel impossible at times. We lack the concentration, inclination and focus to see it through. I always find visuals help me a lot, and try to picture an eye when I close my eyes so that I can concentrate on something, and use it to zone out on. Colour in this eye on the page and then use it to focus on if you feel you need a moment to zone out or meditate.

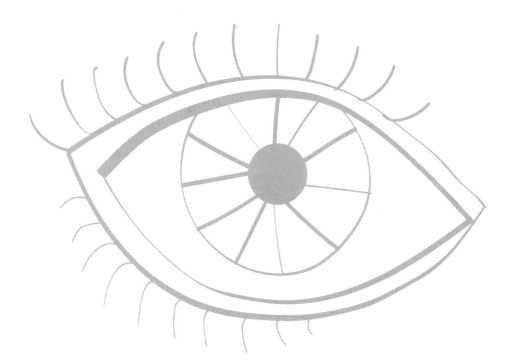

RAINBOWS OF EMOTIONS

All of our moral compasses are set differently and will lean more emphatically towards certain subjects or beliefs than others, proving that a lot of what we vehemently believe to be wrong or right is just our unique vision of the world. Feeling free within the walls of our own concepts and also understanding our own emotional depths are vital to help us to travel towards calm. For example, maybe you feel very stressed when you think you haven't succeeded at work. We have labelled failure or not doing our best as 'wrong'. Well, who made up that rule and why should you believe in it? There is no guarantee that by being the best at something you will feel happier, calmer or more relaxed about life. It's the same with how we label emotions. We have a drawn up list socially that depicts which emotions are positive and which are negative, so when we feel one is on the 'bad' list we tend to layer it up with a heavy dose of stress, too – stress induced by the knowledge that we are dipping into the 'wrong' emotion.

I used to, and sometimes still do, feel sadness is negative. It's a tough thing to admit that you simply feel sad but it is also okay. As soon as we remember that we lose the inner stress of trying to battle it away or store it up physically. I believe it's far better to let that particular emotion flow out of you in any way which feels right, rather than caging it all up to manifest into perhaps intense sadness or even anger later down the line.

So – if you find yourself feeling sad – go for it, listen to sad music and weep in your kitchen, call a friend to tell them you feel vulnerable, wail into your cup of tea on a rainy night. Let it all out until the sorrow has moved through every inch of your body, leaving you revived and most likely rejuvenated. Being sad doesn't have to be a negative experience, it's simply a process of digesting certain moments in your life. Crying is not a sign of weakness, it is simply the quickest and most effective way of moving through emotion. I quite enjoy a good cry these days.

We need to stop labelling emotions as 'right' or 'wrong' and just simply feel what is naturally there. So don't fight it or feel stressed about it, let it flow in and out again and give it the time and attention it deserves. Accepting the whole emotional spectrum allows us to process and let go of what we are digesting throughout our lives. If we know it's okay to 'feel it all' we can approach each emotional state with an underlying calm.

PUTTING OUT THE FIRE

The emotion I personally feel quite conflicted about is feeling angry or simply a bit rotten. It seems like a harder emotion to expel than sorrow. Sadness can flow out with physical tears and heavy sobs that move it all on nicely. At times anger can feel a little scary. Again, I think it's fine to feel anger, to feel passion and rage about a certain injustice or sore point in life, I just don't think it's okay to take it out on others. It's not for them to deal with even if you believe it is. Anger can be a very fiery experience so there's usually a hefty amount of weight behind its impetus. Use this energy wisely to move in the right direction. Anger is there to teach us about our emotions and to help us move on. If this anger has no release and sits in you for an extended period of time,

We all go through a myriad of emotions throughout every day. In one day, we can feel as if the seasons have changed several times before we go to bed because of our emotions. Write down all the emotions you have felt today and the one you are currently feeling; don't be scared to be totally honest and then own it. Accept the emotion, welcome it in but know there's also no need to hold on to it for too long. Imagine it flowing in and out naturally.

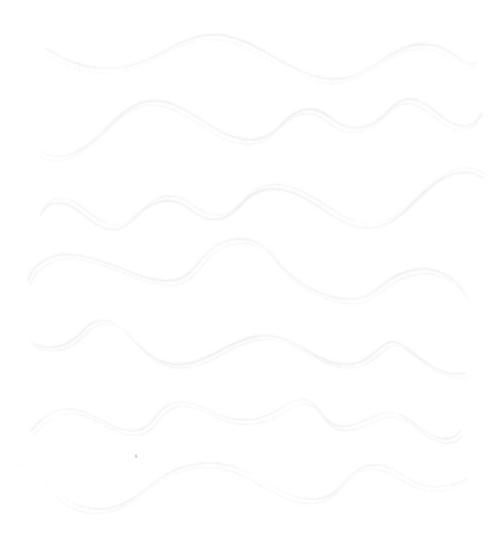

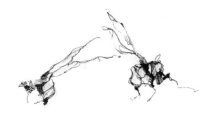

it'll more than likely morph into irritation. It'll feel like a constant itch that lives just beneath the surface of your skin. I've definitely harboured anger related to specific people and situations in my life and they usually physically manifest somewhere down the line. It could be headaches, poor digestion or low immunity, but that anger will try to find a way out somehow. It's always best to let it go when you know deep down you've had enough – know that it serves you no purpose.

I have made many a debatable decision when rage has been in the driving seat. I've had arguments, said things I didn't need to and let it speak instead of my heart. I'm nowhere near mastering this one but I always endeavour to PAUSE before I act. If someone has riled you, ruffled your feathers or caused sparks in your life, you might be feeling desperate to speak out. The fire in your belly creates a surge of energy that needs to be freed. Your heart races, your cheeks flush and you shout and rant about the injustice of it all. In these situations I instantly panic that if I don't have my say then even more boundaries will be crossed and even more injustice will occur. I believe in these volcanic moments that my words can defeat the opposition in one fell swoop.

Does this ever really end well? Not for me! I always regret my actions and wish I had waited before I acted. I now constantly strive to only act once I'm feeling calm. This has taken me a long time to figure out but it was worth the wait, although I'm still working on this one, big time!

If you believe you have suffered injustice and you are still not ready to speak up, try to help yourself by helping others who you believe may have experienced something similar. This action will transfer that inner dormant anger and rage into a potent energy that can do some real good. You could also do something physical to help move this feeling along, like we chatted about in the body chapter.

FIND THE LESSON

It's also completely okay to feel deflated. I've made friends with this one over the years. I've learned that it usually means I need to stop and take a clearer look around me. In these moments I need to take an inventory of what is bringing me down, or I should say, what I'm allowing to bring me down. Taking responsibility for what you're letting in is sometimes half the battle. We can feel deflated because others are attempting to put us down. We let in their negativity or start to believe in others' mistruths about ourselves. We forget the good and only focus on what people are alerting us to.

Our balloon can also burst when we don't feel loved back in equal measure. This is stressful because we then feel needy and slightly desperate as we scramble to love a bit more in the hope we'll see it returned.

We can feel deflated when we feel we haven't done our best. When we know we could have spoken with kinder words, acted more lovingly or just kept quiet. This is when we beat ourselves up somewhat and end up with the wind knocked out of us.

I've had many moments in relationships and in my career where I have felt totally defeated and rock bottom and then spotted a tiny chink of light. At first that feeling is like you've remembered something really great but can't quite place what it is. That feeling is hope and it can be a big enough spark to make you realise that change and newness are possible. Sometimes I only feel defeated because I'm looking around me at everyone else far too intensely. My own story and version of success may differ to others and that comparison makes me believe that I am less than those around me. Classic glass-half-empty stuff. But if I take a step back and stop comparing myself to others I can see with clarity that I'm just taking a different route, rather than failing. Eliminate that stress by remembering that your life and success will be different to that of those around you.

Striving to meet other people's expectations will never make for a calm experience and will muddle your own ideas of what you're looking for in life. One friend might believe that power equals success, whereas your own version of success simply means enjoying what you do. Others may believe that being extremely busy equals success, whereas you may think that having a balance in life feels like the end goal for you. Stick to your own version of what success means and if you do feel deflated, use that moment as a springboard to look for new roads and change. Being deflated can teach us to stop comparing and to also think outside the box. Not such a negative state of mind after all!

AND DON'T FORGET . . .

It's okay to get things wrong sometimes. How on earth are we supposed to learn otherwise? I've made millions of mistakes – I could write the longest list right now of all the terrible decisions I've made, stupid things I've said and moments where I haven't been at my best. This is life. This is the reality of being a human. Social media and our fondness of knowing everyone else's business would have you think otherwise but I'm assuring you now that it is A-okay to balls it up at times. If we were to travel along in life getting everything spot on, acing exams, getting every job we applied for,

Often we feel our stresses are bigger than we are. Use this trick if you're in need of some perspective. In the boxes on the left write a list of all the things you are worried about today. Now imagine yourself a year from now and write down how you'll feel about them then. How many do you think you'll still be worrying about? Concentrate on a solution for those, but use this 'time-machine' power to know the other worries aren't worth it in the bigger picture.

TIME MACHINE

TODAY

A YEAR FROM NOW

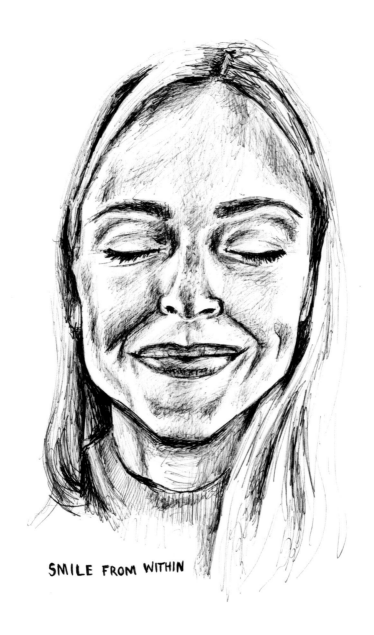

SMILE FROM WITHIN

staying in glowing relationships and friendships forever, we would learn so much less. We wouldn't expand emotionally or be given huge signs to try something new. Of course, when things are going well it feels wonderful, but we all need that balance to make us appreciate, learn and move on to new pastures.

Mistakes can feel overly stressful because other people's opinions about it can be hurtful. This can be an extremely painful process (believe me, I know about that one with my peculiar job) and we have to have ten-tonne strength to block out the loud voices shouting out their penny's worth. This stress is only real if we believe in what others are saying. If we know deep down it is okay to make mistakes and that we shall not be defined by them or other people's opinions, we can start to dissipate stress. I find it very useful to know that every person out there casting judgment has ALSO made mistakes. They're probably only choosing to highlight yours as they believe it may take the heat off their own!

It's okay to feel sad, angry, defeated and as if we've made mistakes, it's how we process these states of mind that counts. Let those emotions flow, don't judge yourself for feeling them, don't hold on to them for extended periods of time and don't pass them on to someone else in a negative way. It's okay to feel how you feel. Accepting all of our varying states with open arms decreases stress immediately as there is no resistance from within. We accept and process and welcome back the calm.

Summary

FIND YOUR SWEET SPOT.

Locate where calm metaphorically sits in your body so you can revisit it always.

FEEL WHAT YOU FEEL.

Don't tell yourself off for your emotions – let them come and go.

VISUALISE.

If you're feeling stressed, picture something to help you bring back the calm.

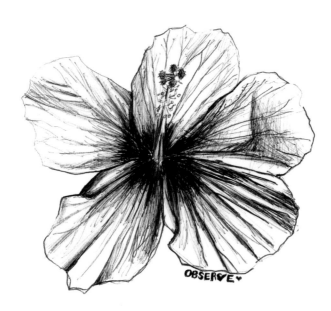

OBSERVE

WHAT DOES A CALM MIND LOOK LIKE TO YOU?

Write one word or draw a picture here that sums it up.

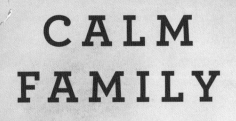

CALM
FAMILY

Family can often be a paradoxical world of calm and chaos.
It can be both the crashing waves on the surface and
the still of the ocean bed, simultaneously. There will be
members of your family who make you feel calm by the
mere mention of their name, but also characters in your
pack who make your muscles tense to think about. Those
who nurture, those who listen, those who think with clarity,
will more than likely be the ones whio you call when in
trouble or turn to when you feel chaotic.

A BIT ABOUT US

In my family my mum offers me so much strength and support but she can also easily get tangled up in fear and worry. Her love for me and my brother is robust and omnipresent but this intensity of emotion, at times, makes her lose her cool. I could fall into her arms at any point and I know they would be outstretched and waiting, but I also know what information I should confide in her and what to leave out. This is the burden of being a mother, as I well know. The thought of your most loved ones being hurt or feeling pain is enough to rock your boat completely.

My dad joins the dots of this family puzzle nicely. He is considered and grounded and seemingly unphased. He isn't unflappable but the circumstances that throw him off are often small nuances rather than catastrophic sagas. For instance, he loves (like I do) to hit the sack early. If he is out and socialising there will be a finite amount of time he is willing to endure being that far away from his comfy bed and if the clock tips past this allotted time he will get flustered. Yet when it comes to drama he takes it all in his stride. He removes his own emotions from the story he is digesting and displays a cool head to offer up advice and unpick the worry, revealing some much-needed clarity. All in all, I feel very lucky to have a strong mother who I can turn to and an unflappable father – as long as you get him home by 10p.m.!

I also feel rather lucky to have a gang of very cool cousins, aunts and uncles. The Cotton side of my family is very laid-back, so my family on this side all walk with an air of calm around them at all times. Their company is light, fun and always good-humoured. My mother's side of the family is all about nurturing. Any member on that side of the family would find it excruciating to visit your home without bringing at least three unexpected gifts. Pot plants, biscuits in ornate tins and small crystals for your handbag. They're the most generous and giving people I've ever met and sweet without the saccharine. They're peaceful people who would jump in front of a bullet for you – whilst clinging onto a house plant.

FAMILY DRAMA

There will more than likely be drama in a corner of your family. Whether close by or not the repercussions will still ricochet through the generations and create questions and, at times, stress. I have experienced this over the years and it can be discombobulating. The roots of your family tree seem to lift from the soil as you feel the generational shift through the branches. Outside of our families, I'm sure we all try to avoid stress-inducing characters, but when we are related by blood, marriage or joined families, it can be beyond testing. It also means you're probably going to be seeing them a fair bit in life; even if geographically there is a distance or boundary, it's hard to cut off all contact with someone in your family.

Even if the contact is minimal, you'll still hear whispers of their actions and possibly feel enraged by this secondhand news. There's no getting away from it. So how do we keep our cool in these situations? How do we avoid getting sucked into the vortex of drama and stress? How do we find the calm?

There is usually someone in a family who knows exactly how to press our buttons. They know you so well they have the ability to tap into areas of yourself others can't. If you can relate to that, write down what buttons are pushed most regularly for you on the calculator below. Acknowledging our weak spots is the first step in learning how to stop them being an issue in the future.

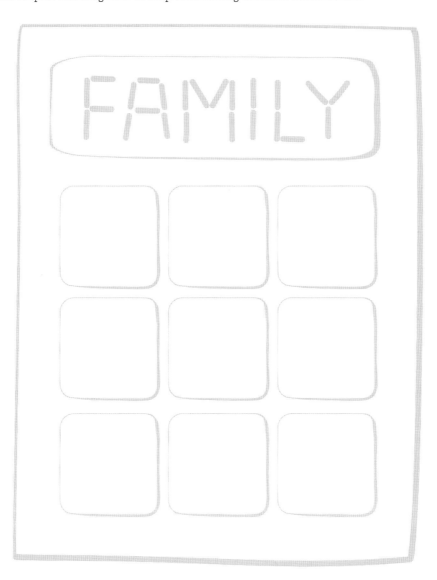

The first thing I try to do is step back. If the drama isn't affecting us directly it's much better to just hear the stories, feel the emotions that naturally rush in with the news and then let it pass. If we know we cannot help the situation and that our being involved will probably only worsen it, we have to step back. It can be so tempting to get sucked into a tasty dose of drama, or to let old wounds reopen, but delving in further rarely ends well. If there's discomfort within your family network and you know you CAN help out, then of course step that bit closer and do what you can. Any stress that seems to attach itself to you in these moments can be somewhat diluted with the knowledge that you're coming at it from a place of love.

I feel constantly inspired by those in my family who take each step thoughtfully and spread calm with a single smile. I try to emulate their actions when I find myself in tricky spots, as naturally I can find it hard to hold my tongue. I've let words tumble out of my mouth before pausing for thought, and of course this has made situations that bit worse. Acting and speaking when you are once again calm is usually the best option. I am still stumbling along with this idea and don't always remember to apply it to my own story, but it's one worth practising.

Sometimes in families you just have to accept there are some members you are not going to get along with so easily, and that is okay. Let antagonists antagonise, let the irresponsible be irresponsible, let the narcissist look only one way. Just get on with your own story when you can and don't bite on the bait that some people offer. Family tension is often that bit more intense than other types, because you care so much. The love is deep, the connection is strong and the loss feels heavier.

'CALM' PARENTING (HA!)

As a mother I'm a confusing combination of calm and chaos. Having children has brought up emotions in me I didn't know existed, as the love I feel is all-consuming and often blinding. Parenting is complex and exhausting as well as life-affirming and intoxicating. In my twenties I started to experience deep swells of broodiness where I dreamed up hazy scenes of me and my flock of five-plus children picnicking in the sunshine. I imagined I would be a super chilled-out and care-free mother who never worried or faltered where her children were concerned.

Cut to me in a dirty tracksuit pleading with my four-year-old to 'JUST TRY ONE PIECE OF BROCCOLI' in a rather desperate tone! Where did that kaftan-wearing, floaty and relaxed mum go? Well, she never existed, because from the second I gave birth the worry wrapped around my bloated postnatal body and has tinkered alongside my intense love for my kids ever since. I'm not sure I've met a mum who is stress- or worry-free. If you are out there please contact me and let me know all your secrets!

The anxiety of parenting starts way before the baby is even born. When you're pregnant you're bombarded with advice and nostalgic comments from others which is hard to process when you're dealing with a sore back, possibly sickness (ME!) and itchy leggings. It is the most exciting time ever but also completely bizarre as it's all the unknown. Here's my own advice on how to stay calm when pregnant: if people genuinely want to offer up a practical note that has helped them through the early days, then maybe jot down their pearls of wisdom, but if someone seems to just be enjoying a nostalgic monologue fired your way, nod, smile and ditch it. It'll be different for you anyway. No pregnancy is the same. My two pregnancies were dramatically different to each other so I couldn't even offer myself advice. Take one day at a time, go with the flow.

Being a parent brings out the very best of you and at times the worst, too. There are days, sometimes weeks, where life with my children flows beautifully. They eat their dinner without complaint; they have a bath without fighting over the same rubber duck, and they go to bed after two short stories they've heard a million times. I go to bed feeling happy, relaxed and . . . yes . . . CALM! These moments are golden and precious and probably the only ones I'll choose to recall at a later date when they're all big and grown up.

MY 'MUM WORRIES'

Then there are the days, or indeed weeks, where I am walking through treacle. Every part of the day is a battle and all aspirations of iPad-free dinners and bribe-free bedtimes go flying out the window before you can say 'Peppa Pig'. In these moments of pure chaos I usually lose my calm. I'm currently in the epicentre of parenting chaos as both of my children are under five. I do believe, and hope it's not just hearsay, that things do get a little calmer with time and age. It feels like a far-off place for me at the moment but I hold that thought close when having a plate of pasta hurled my way at tea time. I usually have an inner dialogue rolling in these moments that is as confusing and chaotic as my children's behaviour. It starts with

'Be disciplined, otherwise they'll never learn. Stick to the message and the rules you've set out or they'll turn into monsters'.

After half an hour of zero progress my inner mum voice says 'Look . . . pick your battles. Make your life easy and just give him the bloody meringue. I know he's already had a slice of cake today and a meringue is 99 per cent sugar, but hey, you grew up in the 80s when that would have made up one of your five a day'.

This is where it gets confusing. My inner voices start to battle each other, which just adds another heap of chaos to the tornado that's ensuing in my house. I've lost it; my cool AND my calm. It's gone. This is usually when I turn into shouty mum. She's not a part of me I like very much at all, but she is there. Not every day, sometimes she'll be absent for months, but she definitely lurks beneath in times of weakness. I try so hard not to but this internal and external battle seems too much, and when it's topped up with sleep deprivation the cracks begin to show. It's probably the area of calm I'm trying to work on the most. I'm finding it a little easier as time goes on, as I know that shouting or losing my cool will only feed the beast further. My kids pick up on the stress I'm feeling and then behave even worse. What I try to do is remember that I'm feeling so intensely about the situation because I love them so much. This love gets knotted up in frustration and confusion because I want them to have a great life. I want them to eat well, sleep well, behave nicely and have fun, so anything that means we are veering off this path makes me feel like I've not done my best.

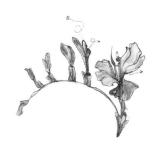

HELLO TO . . . HEIDI

When I am having a mum meltdown I grab my phone with a spag bol covered hand and clumsily type an SOS type message to my dear friend Heidi. In these moments you need solace, recognition and a calm listening ear.

I first met Heidi six years ago, before I had kids myself. Our husbands play in a band together so we were both at the same gig watching from a crowded balcony. I had recently dyed my hair pink, was slightly tipsy on gin and therefore probably quite loud. I'm pretty sure Heidi's first impression of me was not too favourable but luckily she looked past this inebriated inaugural meet and gave me another chance. At this point Heidi was a mum of four and was working on a film she had single-handedly written, produced and directed. To say I was in awe of her energy, work ethic and family values is an understatement. I, on the other hand, was struggling to juggle my career and two cats.

A little further down the line and after having my own children, our friendship has strengthened and comes with an unspoken understanding of life and balance. We both love being mums to our respective children (Heidi went on to have a fifth, who is my gorgeous godson, Sonny) yet fizz with excitement about our creative careers. Juggling these parts of our lives is a constant challenge and one that we love to discuss. When I say 'discuss', it is, more often than not, me pining for seasoned advice, but nonetheless we riff around this subject continuously.

Heidi's down-to-earth approach to life complements her pin-sharp, non-stop creative brain. Her chosen industry of film isn't always female-skewed, so she has had to work relentlessly to fight her corner and get her ideas out there and remains the most relaxed mother I've ever met. I'm still not sure how she cooks for and organises five children on top of her career but she somehow finds a way, whether it's breastfeeding whilst writing up scripts, taking meetings after a complicated morning of getting five kids to various schools or battling on with an inconsistent freelance job knowing that she and her husband have a large family to look after. She is my 'go-to' for family advice and always the most level-headed yet witty person for a good chat, moan or laugh. Her kids all happen to be unbelievably polite and well-mannered, too. After her eldest, Louis, first came to stay with me and my husband, he wrote me a thank-you note! Heaven.

Whatever Heidi is doing, she is doing it right. I'm forever eager to find out more about her family alchemy and personal aptitude for juggling life, so I took this book as an opportunity to quiz her further.

F: You are one of my mum heroes and I am in constant wonder as to how you make the cogs of family life keep turning. What makes you lose your calm?

H: I am quite calm these days, but I haven't always been this way. I suppose the change came from making a decision to embrace the chaos instead of fighting it. The one thing that still manages to make me lose my calm is when others affect my work running smoothly. I have to run such a tight ship to be able to do what I do and take care of my family simultaneously, so if it is rocked it still gets my goat. At these times I have to try to remember that you can't control everything and sometimes you have to trust and let it go. One of my best friends (you) once told me, 'Just remember, Heidi, the cream always rises to the top' – I take that with me wherever I go.

F: You have five kids and a flying career. When things feel overwhelming and the noise of life is omnipresent, how do you keep cool?

H: I am still working on that. I come from a long line of professional hot heads; I am related to a gangster who was famously shot by the Kray twins for not keeping his cool, for God's sake. When the external or internal noise is too much I go for a run, walk, do yoga – as long as it involves moving outside, preferably with my dogs by my side, it's an instant tonic for me. My husband is great at reminding me what is important. Just after we met, my pancreas decided to turn on itself. Whilst in the hospital the doctors performed a scan and told me, 'Congratulations, you are pregnant. Unfortunately you need major surgery now or you will die. There is very little chance your baby will survive the operation.' That baby is now 16.

F: Do you think it's important to have time for you when you can just focus on being a woman rather than a mother, writer, wife or friend?

H: The times I have felt most focused on being a woman is when I am fully immersed as a mother, writer, wife, friend. When I had my last baby I loved giving myself entirely to him and his brothers and sister, knowing nothing else was more important at that time and that everything else would, and could, wait. This felt empowering. I think sometimes women feel that their other commitments can't afford them this time but it's important to remember that you are allowed to make that choice, and when you do it feels good because you stop the juggling and just enjoy. My girlfriends mean a lot to me, with regards to my focus on being a woman living in the 21st century. Right now I don't have time for hairdos, unless it involves the nit comb.

F: Your job is of a very creative nature. Do you need to be in a calm headspace to get the best out of yourself?

H: Yes. If I go onto a set with a hot head two things would happen. Number one, it would spread amongst the cast and crew like wildfire. The director starts shouting and screaming and suddenly everyone is at each other's throats and nothing is achieved. Number two, everyone would think I was a complete tosser and no one would listen to me. I am so grateful to do what I love, I am always calm on set because I am genuinely so happy to be there.

F: How do you manage to keep on top of all your children's lives, activities and needs, and does it ever feel too much?

H: With five kids from one to 16 the most challenging aspect is spotting their different needs as they arise. Kids don't always tell you the stuff they really need so you have to pay attention. I have to check myself sometimes and make sure that I have spent time with every one of them at some point every day, even if it's just on the phone if I'm not at home. The only time it ever feels too much is when I get out of the bath and have to dry myself on a face cloth because they have used all the towels.

F: How do you find your calm in the chaos of life? Is it an activity? A headspace? A person?

H: I write scripts, immersing myself in imaginary worlds with imaginary people, and I swear that this is what keeps me sane. On the other hand, it could be the reason behind my madness, let's not analyse it too much! I also listen to loud music and dance with the kids. Right now we are learning to dance like Michael Jackson, it's very therapeutic.

F: Can you recall a particular moment of bliss in your life where everything felt serene and calm?

H: After a birthday dinner in Sardinia with my husband, my kids and friends, we went swimming in the sea as the sun went down and I remember feeling truly at peace. Calm moments are very few and far between, but I don't think we should worry too much about that. Often the things that drive us and make us the people we want to be are not born out of calm, but out of complete chaos.

"

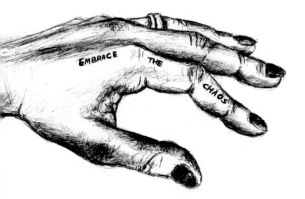

MUM DOUBT

Being a mother drives self-doubt screeching into the limelight, which is so draining when you're already dealing with everyday chaos. You compare yourself to others, forget all the good that you do and beat yourself up when things don't go to plan. Stepping back from the situation and taking a moment to remember the good you've done, the hard work you've put into the family and the love that you hold, can at times be enough to bring it all back to calm. Not always instantly, of course, but it'll certainly help.

This usually leads me to either ignoring the tantrum that's raging on, which in turn defuses it in time, or allows me the patience to sit and talk a little more softly and with a little more understanding to try to get my kids on the same page as me. This sometimes works and sometimes doesn't, but at least I know 'this all too shall pass' and we'll have one of those glorious calm days again soon. Believe me, I'm working on this one all the time, but I do believe that talking honestly about this to each other helps other parents feel less alone in it all.

Being a parent is a chance to learn a lot about ourselves. I know that I get panicky when we slip out of our usual family routine and feel extremely tense when my kids seem unhappy. I forget to trust in life and need to remind myself that I have to allow my children to learn about life's ups and downs without my constant protection. This in turn reminds me how unsettled I can feel when things don't turn out as I had imagined in my own life. These moments are a mirror being held back up to us, if we choose to see it in this way.

Don't forget, we are also one of the first few generations trying to do it all. We want to be the best parents we can be, the best at work, organised and on top of everything that's going on. These demands that we place on ourselves can strip away the calm quite quickly, leaving us exasperated. Remembering that we don't have to BE it all is vital if we want to basically just stay sane.

Sometimes it can be helpful to write down exactly what you believe a good mum is. Make a list of all the specifications you believe a 'good' mum should have then look back over it and realise you're doing most of it anyway! Parenting is chaos, and you can learn to embrace some of that; finding our calm in it all is optional and challenging, but probably always a great idea for our own sanity!

METHOD IN THE MADNESS

I'm also a step-parent, which I am very proud of and grateful for. I'm very lucky that my step-kids are extremely cool – and very calm to boot. They bring very little chaos to the party and for that I'm even more thankful. My step-daughter is one of the few people on this planet who can bring my son Rex out of an earth-shattering tantrum. She'll distract him with a silly face or story and the next thing you know he's laughing his head off and miraculously has turned back into an angel child. She is able to click into his sense of humour and wavelength in a way that I'm not always capable of, as I'm bogged down with the pragmatic side of family life.

Sometimes I get very bogged down with worry that I'm not a good enough mum. I have chosen to go back to on/off work and with that often comes a whole heap of guilt. I know deep down I'm doing my best but sometimes a more obvious reminder is needed. This is when my favourite hobby of list writing comes in very handy! I write down all the things I believe a good mum should be. Then when I look back over the list I realise they're attributes I already have. We tend to over-complicate what we believe our roles should be so this activity can bring a certain clarity. Whatever title you think of yourself as most – whether that's a mum or a brother or a daughter or a friend – write a list here of what you consider the best version of that person to be, and then look back and see how many of these specifications you're already hitting up!

....

....

....

....

....

....

....

....

....

The only chaos that comes with having all four kids in the house is the militant organisation that my husband and I have to adhere to if we want things to run smoothly. We battle chaos with one mighty swipe of nerdy organisation. Weekend sports activities to remember, lifts to certain social engagements, homework reminders, six loads of washing, staggered meal times due to schedules... oh, and remembering to have some fun along the way.

By default I slip into this 'organising mode' when things feel out of line. It makes me feel instantly calmer when I feel in control, but I have the habit of letting this not only defuse impending anarchy but also reducing the FUN! Those lists and delegated orders suffocate fun in seconds and life becomes played out rather than lived. My husband is always the one to remind me of these pitfalls and drags me kicking and screaming out of my notebook and back into the living. There is room for it all. Making lists and getting things organised brings me a sense of calm that I can't find in many other places with a family of our size, but I have to get the balance right and not turn into Mrs Boring from List Land. Again, it's something I'm working on.

Chaos and calm will look very different to us all where family is concerned. No matter how packed or chilled your own household is there will be stresses and chaos and you will develop your own methods of relieving it all.

Over the last six and a half years since becoming a step-parent and parent, I have worked out that I can use my methods of taming the unruly to bring some calm but I must remember to have fun along the way. I can dish out a bit of rigidity when needed but I also must let go so that life can show me new lessons. I can write lists and try to make sense of the volume of needs in our house but I must stop to smell the coffee en route. I must also remember the chaos will pass. It always does.

I think the same goes for those of us in a marriage or partnership. If you are married, living with a life partner or cohabiting with mates there has to be a balance of chaos and calm. We all have very different needs at home and finding meet-in-the-middle moments is vital.

MEETING IN THE MIDDLE

Consideration. A word I hadn't given any thought to in my teens and early twenties. I moved out of my parents' house at 19 and lived alone doing as I pleased. I ate what I wanted, when I wanted. I kept my flat as tidy or unkempt as I so chose and I sang loudly at any time of day I desired. Living with someone makes you rethink all your own personal habits and quirks and makes theirs stand out in a toe-curling manner. An ex-boyfriend of mine got pretty irate when I had not put all of his shower gels and shampoos 'label facing out' after I had taken my morning wash. This was not a procedure I was used to or could have given a toss about, but I quickly became aware of this ritual's great importance to him. Suffice to say, things didn't work out with that one, but even now my beloved husband and I have habits that annoy the shit out of each other and make our worlds slightly less calm in the process.

I am a neat freak. When my husband leaves cupboard doors open after he's made a cup of tea, I want to throw every single teabag onto the street in a fit of rage. Equally my need for order is increasingly frustrating for Jesse, when I hang up clothes he has only seconds before got out of the wardrobe to put on. We piss each other off in so many little ways but by understanding our own needs and beliefs we can both let go a little and not let it all build up.

I think delegating is awfully important in shared homes, too. I am useless at asking for help as I'm fiercely independent but I have learned over the years that it only gets me in more of a mess and leads to more stress if I try to do too much. That's not very helpful to me or anyone else for that matter. My husband happens to be a very helpful fellow so he is happy to pick up the parts of life I sometimes feel overwhelmed with. This leads to a very cooperative partnership when it comes to household stuff and bringing up our kids. If things feel off balance your end with your partner in life or friend you live with, make sure you're honest and that you're sharing the responsibilities in your home, so you can get that calm in your relationship. It can be tough to be honest as far as help and change are concerned, but those hard-to-say words are much more preferable than sinking into resentment and a whole host of other emotions that will cause a lot of stress and very little calm.

It is very easy to react without thinking when family members push our buttons. Taking stock of how we react and looking for patterns helps us try to change our thought process and reactions. Complete the following sentences.

Sometimes .... breaks my calm. When he/she does

....

I behave in this way: ....

....

....

I know I don't have the power to change them, so instead I can react in this way:

....

....

.... which will bring calm back into my life.

CRAZY IN LOVE

Now on to something more fun: falling in love. I'm not sure many relationships start out in a calm way and I think most of us are okay with that. Most relationships start in a frenzy of intense emotion and complete chaos. Sweet joyful chaos. A bit like the Big Bang! Particles bash and crash against each other, ricocheting around like balls in a pinball machine. Electric energy runs the show as pupils dilate and hearts beat a little faster. Nothing about falling in love feels calm. How can it when it is all so new, exciting and unknown? There are no guarantees and no plan in place, it is simply exquisite free-falling with a huge grin on your face. I love this part of a relationship, especially the first six months after my husband and I met. All other cares in life seem to fly out of the window that's been left open on a hazy summer afternoon. Wine, late nights and flushed red cheeks replace the humdrum thoughts about post that you know needs opening, being punctual for appointments and everyday stress. It's the one time when most of us can properly let go.

Falling in love requires true vulnerability as it's stepping into the complete unknown. If you've been hurt before and feel stressed about falling for someone else, take it from me – who has been hurt many a time over the years – it's so worth taking the chance again. Finding calm in this romantic whirlwind seems far less urgent. There may be the odd moment of pining for the security of cohabiting or marriage as you try to fast-forward time, but really just try to enjoy the vortex of intensity and love you're experiencing before all of that comes. You may feel a slight stress in the uncertainty of new love but not even marriage and kids can secure that, so just go with it – find a chunk of calm on this love waltzer ride by simply sitting in the moment. Allow the adrenaline and new emotional brevity to whirl around you. Be comfortable in the chaos, that's how you'll find calm.

FIRST DATE PANIC

I couldn't NOT write about this. Is there any moment more un-calm than a first date? The day of my first official date with my now-husband was a sweat-drenched, slow-motion day. The clock ticked so slowly to reach 7p.m., the time when we would meet. I flapped around my house feeling completely deranged and then thought I would go and bug one of my mates down the road instead. I couldn't sit in this feeling of excited chaos on my own for a second longer. My friend Richard is a bit of an expert on love and relationships as he writes about the subject and also has a long-term relationship and four kids. He instantly calmed me by reminding me that it's great to embrace this chaos. It's the sort of inner anarchy that makes you see everything with new eyes. It lights up each cell in your body and allows you to take a chance and be a little reckless, in a good way. Another pearl of wisdom he imparted is one I've since passed on to many friends. I had asked him what the hell I should wear to impress and he told me to stick with what I was wearing already. He told me that on that first date, you should wear the exact clothes that you were wearing when your suitor texted you or called to ask you out (unless you were in your pyjamas or happened to be at an 80s fancy-dress party!).

At that moment I had on a George Michael T-shirt and a skirt that felt a little under-dressed, but Richard assured me this was the exact laid-back look I was after. I just hoped Jesse liked Wham! as much as I did! This nugget of advice, I guess, really just means BE YOU! Don't dress up any differently or act any differently to how you would when with a mate. Don't hide behind how you think they want you to be – be you, be relaxed and calm being yourself. I can't fully hold Richard responsible for the following seven years of union including three years of marriage, but I can certainly appreciate his wisdom which helped me through that initial frenzy of dating emotions. Thanks, Richard!

FINDING OUR OWN CALM

Some people out there are addicted to those crazed feelings at the start of a new relationship and find it hard to move past this point. Perhaps they assume things get boring after a while and don't give longevity a chance. I love that first frenzied period but I wouldn't swap it for the comfort and rhythm that I have in life now. I love the calm that surrounds my union with my husband. It's one we chose to honour in marriage –which might not be for everyone, but for us felt like it solidified our choices in life. Our life might not be raucous, with late nights and spontaneous trips to the tattoo parlour so much these days, but it is still loads of fun. We laugh more than ever, we venture further into our journey of learning together as we raise our children, and we help each other out. These are the things that matter to us and our family unit, and they are the parts of our life that we put an enormous amount of energy into. We now get our kicks from family life, stolen moments as a couple, the love we get from our kids and all the chaos that our life all together brings.

Stress and calm are inevitably threaded throughout the entire journey from new love, to marriage, to procreating, to death or divorce. Life is an unknown and we'll deal with situations as they arise. No relationship is perfect and none is without its stresses. For me, it's about trying not to let everyday stress overshadow the deep love that we all have for each other in our family – and also remembering that it is okay to relax in the calm moments when they arise.

THE CIRCLE OF LIFE

The acknowledgment that there will be lots of ups and downs in our relationships as life continues to throw change at us can perhaps also be applied to how we look at life more generally. We will all experience stress in different ways throughout our lifetimes and to varying degrees, but we all share a common ground: change. Change can be positive and enlightening but also very stressful and complicated.

The first time the majority of us experience stress is during our teen years. CHANGE! It's everywhere. Our bodies morphing before our very eyes as our minds try to keep up with the pace at which we hurtle towards adulthood. We are not young enough to be free in our bodies as we were in childhood but not comfy in our new adult skin to truly feel okay. It can be very exciting and intoxicating, yet this limbo-land can

One way of diluting stress and rage when someone in your family is frustrating you is to put yourself in their shoes. Think more deeply about why they are acting in a certain way and try to think about what is causing them to do so. In the first shoe write down the family member and their actions and in the second shoe write down the real reasons you think they're doing it.

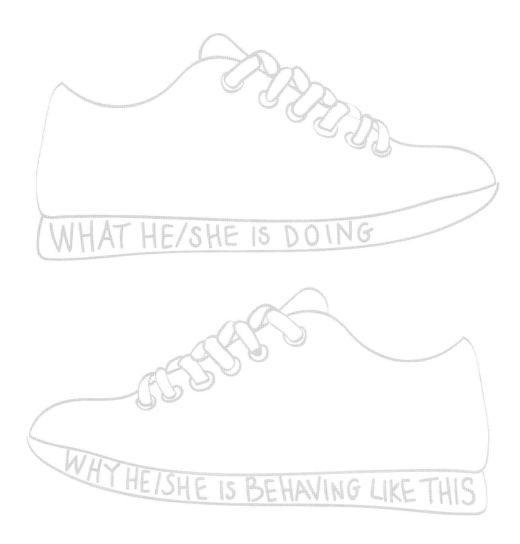

WHAT HE/SHE IS DOING

WHY HE/SHE IS BEHAVING LIKE THIS

also be stressful. During our teen years we also try to figure out what relationships mean for the first time whilst navigating through the options that could lead us to who and where we want to be in the world. Suddenly, responsibility and organisation seem scary and very real.

Next up we are faced with the change that relationships carry, such as cohabiting, compromising and learning to trust someone outside of our family life as they become a new wing of our tribe. This can add layers of support that we hadn't previously known, but this change can also feel overwhelming and possibly stressful too. Then perhaps you move on to parenthood or a career, or maybe both. More compromise and a whole new value placed on your time arrives, which can present a lot of anxiety as well as personal expansion.

And then we have to get our heads around ageing, with its bone-creaking trepidation and wrinkled-foreheaded worry. This is a time to perhaps change our pace in life and celebrate so much, but it is also certainly rife with change.

Change is certain, stress is probable, but joy is also everywhere if you look for it. It's funny how, in this neverending cycle of life, change and death is discombobulating even though we know it is 100 per cent normal. It's how it's been for thousands of years and will continue to be for a long time from now, yet we still feel the tremor of fear and uncertainty around them. Maybe that's all part of it. These shake-ups in life present us with lessons which can be bitten off with a tense jaw and a heap of stress or with a huge sense of letting go. When I last saw my 94-year-old great-uncle Hadyn (who I'm so pleased featured in *HAPPY*) he said quite casually, 'do come and see me before I pop off'. Death to him is perhaps a more easily accepted fate – at 94, perhaps our understanding and willingness to surrender to this inevitable outcome is easier, strengthened with age and wisdom. Perhaps this enlightenment can only be reached after many decades filled with laughter, loss and love?

Although the older generation may be slightly more at peace with their own destiny, for those left behind it can cause a lot of heartache and stress. When my grandparents passed away I felt huge heavy holes open up where their love and character had previously lived, and I can't imagine what it must be like for people who have lost partners, parents or children before their time. This sort of change is heavy and the loss strips away calm as it feels like a building block in your foundations is now missing. Loss can create a lot of chaos, so perhaps rather than desperately scrambling for calm we just need to try to accept it. Understanding that the calm will come back, whilst sitting in the storm of loss, might be the only option we have. If we try to numb the chaos by suppressing our feelings, distracting ourselves or ignoring it altogether it'll more than likely surface at another time. I believe in these darker times we have to try to make peace with chaos whilst remembering the calm will come back at some point down the line.

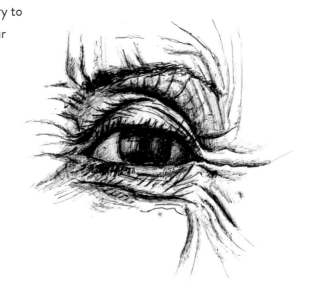

TIME HEALS

We are always going to be faced with change within family life, so in order to find calm we need to decide – do we rail against it, hold our breath and dive into stress? Or do we watch it occur and let go, let it happen and move with it? That is up to each and every one of us. Embracing change will give us a much better chance to either accept the chaos it brings, or find our calm within it.

Summary

STEP BACK.

Respond to any family drama from a calm place.

IF YOU'RE A MUM . . .

. . . accept the chaos! Stop trying to fight it and embrace it instead.

RELAX.

Don't let control get in the way of fun.

WHAT DOES A CALM FAMILY LOOK LIKE TO YOU?

Write one word or draw a picture here that sums it up.

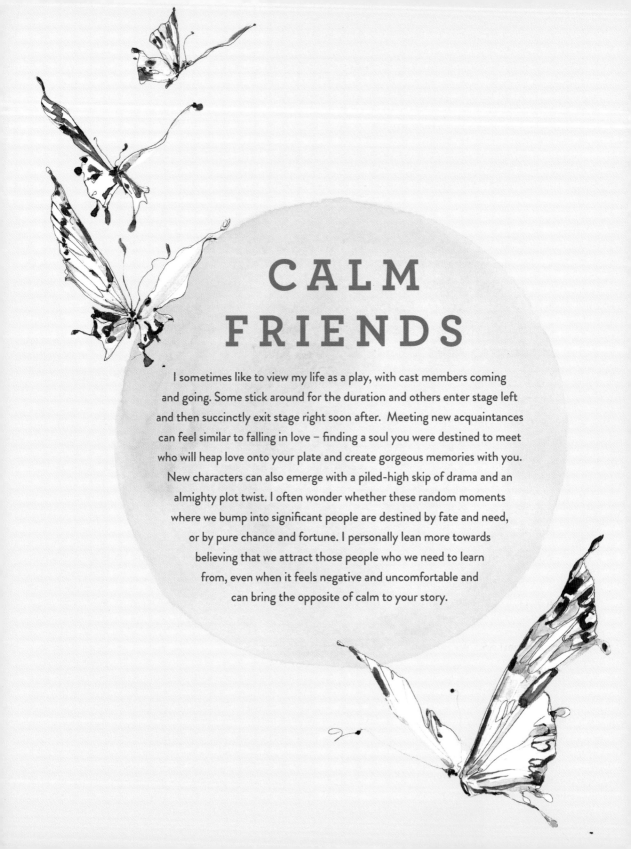

CALM FRIENDS

I sometimes like to view my life as a play, with cast members coming and going. Some stick around for the duration and others enter stage left and then succinctly exit stage right soon after. Meeting new acquaintances can feel similar to falling in love – finding a soul you were destined to meet who will heap love onto your plate and create gorgeous memories with you. New characters can also emerge with a piled-high skip of drama and an almighty plot twist. I often wonder whether these random moments where we bump into significant people are destined by fate and need, or by pure chance and fortune. I personally lean more towards believing that we attract those people who we need to learn from, even when it feels negative and uncomfortable and can bring the opposite of calm to your story.

CALM TYPES

Let's begin with the good stuff! Those people who reduce the heat in those moments of sheer panic and worry. Do you have one of those delightful types in your life who you know will unburden you from your non-stop mind? Isn't it remarkable how another's soothing words have the power to mitigate stress and gain clarity? I feel fit to burst with gratitude that I have some calm warriors in my friendship circle. Did I attract these people into my life to teach me the way, or was it sheer coincidence that they showed up at the right time? I'll never know but I love the magic that emanates from them.

The mere reminder of this web of friendship settles me into a calmer state behind the scenes. If I am going through a patch of drama I know I can call up or email one of these dreamboats, lay myself bare on the table and then receive some much-needed guidance. It's a fresh set of eyes, a new open mind and years of their own experience that can broaden our horizons. That's the first step in reacting in the best way possible. Always use those calm people in your life as a sounding board before you jump into the deep end without your goggles on! Let them see your situation with clarity and let them help you clear the red mist before you react. It may be one simple sentence that acts as the biggest game changer. I always think, 'If I can't see the reality of this situation alone I must ask another around me who can bring the calm'. Opening up your heart and also your ears can be incredibly powerful.

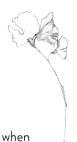

My husband Jesse is 98 per cent calm. It takes a lot to rile him, and even when his personal bees nest is disturbed by another, he deals with it in the most dignified and grounded way. I, unfortunately, do not embody these qualities, so I have to look to him quite regularly for the appropriate way to go about my business. I am like a disgruntled teenager when it comes to reacting to those around me who push my buttons. When someone else's words, actions or opinions challenge my own I can, at times, rise up like a boa constrictor who has been poked with a stick. Calm evaporates in seconds, leaving me in a heap of red-blooded rage. I seem to have to relearn this lesson again and again. I try quickly to look to those calm types in my own life to remind me about the laws of consequence. It's rarely what is going on around us that counts but HOW we react to it.

BEING A CALM TYPE

I feel completely jackpot lucky to have had my own worries and problems somewhat mitigated by people I love and hope to offer the same level of serenity back. The slightly trickier issue is when you're invested in a friend but can't seem to get through to them. You reiterate and recalibrate their dilemma but to no avail. This can in turn rattle your own levels of calm as you feel the situation is exasperated to the max.

Having great mates is a total gift and something I never take for granted! I love my mates and thank the universe for them every day! Make this your friend gratitude page. Stick a photo of your best mates here and celebrate what they bring you in life.

It can be frustrating when someone you love won't listen to your views on a matter that is troubling them but you have to remind yourself that sometimes they are not really ready to let go and start again.

I have had people in my life who seem stuck and I too have been in this predicament many a time. If I'm really honest, there are still a couple of moans that I need to let go of – situations in life that I cannot change but refuse to personally budge opinion so I'm continuously moaning about the same problem. In my twenties a few friends endured my moans about certain situations in life, and although I was besieged with advice and love I still rumbled along without change or action. Hindsight allows me to see their loving point of view and how they were trying to gently lead me out of the stressful situation to the calm, but sometimes when you're in the eye of the storm it takes a long while to figure it all out.

If you know someone who comes to you with the same problem perhaps the friend in question isn't ready to make great leaps, or perhaps they're frightened of leaving their comfort zone. In these situations there is only so much you can do. None of us have the power to make anyone do something they don't want to. We can only hand out kind words from the heart, generate some of our time for them and let them decide on the rest.

It may be testing to be presented with the same problem repeatedly but it's an opportunity for us to learn from it all, too. Why is your friend's suffering causing you irritation and lack of patience? Do we see a little of our own story wrapped up in theirs?

If you are the one who is stuck rigidly in a spot that is making you unhappy, try to route down in to why you aren't making those changes. Are you accepting chaos over calm because that is what you're used to? Or because you think you deserve nothing better?

I felt trapped in work and life situations in my twenties and did my fair share of moaning, and in hindsight I can see I was addicted to that level of drama wherever I went. I wanted to be in the fast lane but couldn't keep up with the speed, so I would fall behind and shout and wail. It didn't cross my mind to try another way until I reached my thirties, when I started to iron out the creases and move at a slightly slower pace. There are still creases galore but I'm much more aware of why they're there. I'm so grateful for my friends who gave such solid advice along the way, although I emphatically ignored it. In retrospect I can see why I did this. I was scared of change. Deep down I knew some of their words were completely true, but to accept what they were saying and to make suggested changes scared the hell out of me. I didn't feel able to slow down with work or lose people from my story who were dragging me down. The responsibility of these decisions felt overwhelming, so it was easier to plod along in the same way and just moan some more.

Not every bit of advice from friends will be right for us, but if deep down you have an inkling that your friends' words can get you out of a stressful situation, perhaps try to swipe fear to one side and make a change knowing you're supported by great mates along the way.

HELLO TO . . . REGGIE

One friend I constantly turn to for life chats and good old-fashioned advice is Reggie Yates. My first memory of Reggie is seeped in kindness. I was 15, extremely professionally inexperienced and in wonder of it all. My first ever TV link to camera was with dear Reggie who calmed my nerves and put a big smile on my face. Even now, one look at Reggie's beaming grin with white gnashers on display is enough to make all my problems fade away.

So back to the echoing TV studio, cameras on and crew at the ready. With nerves fully in the driving seat I cocked up my first piece to camera and then stage whispered 'OH SHIT' which warranted a swift telling off from the director. I thought I had ruined my TV career before reaching the end of my first taped sentence.

Take TWO. Reggie started and fluffed his lines and quietly sighed 'OH shit' feigning complacence and making me feel a whole lot calmer. Reggie's faux mess-up made me look less awful and him appear more human to a nervous me.

This is where our friendship was formed – in one chivalrous move to dilute my own shame and embarrassment. This is pretty much how our relationship has continued, with love, care and humour. Reggie has made me laugh to the point of incontinence and has calmed so many worried and wired moments. It's been a friendship of 20 years that I hope will carry on for many more. I feel unbelievably lucky, and it brings so much calm and support to my life.

F: Hey Reggie. What do you remember about the early days of our friendship?

R: *The Disney Club* feels like five lifetimes ago, when we had the pleasure of sharing with the great British public probably the most awkward stage of our lives, our teens. When we first met, I was maybe 13 or 14 and had already shot a couple of series with the same crew. That continuity helped me feel comfortable on camera and confident in doing what I saw as the most grown-up bit of the day, the work.

At that stage, what interested me almost as much as interviewing pop stars was the shenanigans off set. *The Disney Club* was special as it was a pack of kids hosting a show that somehow wasn't a disaster. To this day I'll never know how you walked into a pack of spotty, hormonal and loud plonkers without even breaking a sweat. You were the new girl who wouldn't take any crap and I loved it. Growing up in a house full of women, my four sisters quickly taught me the type of girl you don't mess with and you filled the criteria. You instantly reminded me of my family, which is probably why to this day I still refer to you as Sis. I'd rip the piss out of your Spice Girl Buffalo trainers and you'd kill me for coming out of the dressing room reeking of Lynx Africa deodorant. I remember you feeling part of the TV family very quickly and that sibling-like connection hasn't changed to this day.

F: I love that you always have time for me and are a brilliant listener, that we can chat passionately about everything from house decor to heartbreak and you never judge or jump to assumptions. What do you get from our friendship?

R: The best relationships I have are built on a similar world view or level of understanding. As I've developed, the importance of emotional intelligence has almost taken pole position in what I look for in any relationship, be it professional, platonic or romantic. Shared experience, albeit bonding, isn't enough to healthily sustain any relationship for two decades. Our friendship, I feel, has lasted due to its foundations.

When we met, we both knew that the job we were doing could be taken away at any time. That understanding changed our behaviour and relationship with money, fame and the job in exactly the same way. Whenever I looked at how you saw the world, it married with my value system which told me I could trust you in an environment full of shallow and at times bloody scary people.

I've never asked myself what I get from any friendship because I honestly don't have many new ones. Those whom I call friends have grown with me and I think as we've become adults our tastes in footwear and deodorant may have changed, but our values haven't.

F: What do you think makes a solid friendship and does a good one bring calm?

R: As I've always had a complicated relationship with my actual family, I see friends as the family you choose. Moving out at 18 and fighting for my own sense of independence, the people I turned to for help or advice usually weren't blood.

Trust and honesty for better or worse live as the backbone to everything I have of value in my life, especially my friendships.

F: How hard do you think it is to give a friend honest advice, especially if it may not be the answer they're looking for?

R: I spent years doing what I was told professionally while ignoring what I felt. The minute I gained a level of confidence in my gut, taste and opinion, my entire career changed for the better.

I avoid like the plague receiving advice from people who haven't lived or experienced the thing they claim to be an expert about. So when it comes to the people I love and sharing with them my take on any given situation, I try to see their issue through the lens of an experience of my own. It can be challenging, but I have to be honest with friends and myself if they come to me for help. There's nothing worse than the friend who says 'I told you so' – when they never actually did!

F: I love how calming it can be to meet face to face with someone and really connect. Chatting and switching up ideas feels important. How important do you think it is to make an effort and put physical face time into the equation?

R: Face time with friends I find essential. It may sound super Maya Angelou, but that shit is soul food to me! I go as far as looking at my calendar months in advance and planning out days where friends and I can go for dinner or drinks.

I spent years working on myself and what I could be doing to be a better man, but the minute everything clicked into place was when I realised it's not actually about me. Investing in people is one of the most important things in my life and that investment, I feel, is just as important with friends and strangers.

To allow a busy schedule to prevent investing in the right things just isn't good enough. To make time for a friend to simply ask whether they're okay is so important, as we all need to unpack and learn with people we can trust.

Since making the effort to give my energy to people or the issues I care about, I've felt nothing but support from friends and family without even asking for it. That return I don't see as being out of obligation – I honestly believe that's how things work.

"

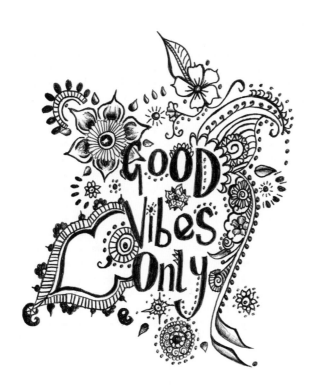

When acquaintances and people in our lives bring us down, feel toxic, or make us react in a certain way it is good to have a list of rules to try and stick to. This always helps me when I'm navigating confrontation or am trying to defer drama. Mine go a little something like this:

- *I will not talk about the person in question.*

- *I will not allow them to take away my happiness.*

- *I will not feel fear around them or worry what they can take from me.*

- *I will fill my heart with those I love instead.*

I will then look back to this in times of need. Write below your own list of rules and when you feel you need them refer to this book or take a photo of them on your phone so they're always close by.

....

....

....

....

....

....

....

....

HELLO TO . . . BONNY

One of my great friends, Bonny, is different to me in so many ways, yet the magic is there, woven through each of our emails to one another that fly across the ocean that parts us. When we see each other, once or twice a year, our friendship is bound even tighter, with more memories made and more stories told.

Bonny Kinloch was born in 1943 in China, the youngest person to enter the Lunghua Japanese prison camp. Her story began in unusual circumstances, but her life continued in this vivid, unique way. Bonny now resides in Ibiza and has called it home since 1979. She is now 26 years old – at every birthday since she turned 50 she has decided to count backwards. This is one of the many things I love about her.

I first met dear Bon Bon five years ago , when my husband and I were on a summer holiday in Ibiza. I had at this point already been told many a tale about this eccentric and magical lady who was Jesse's late mother's best friend. Jesse thinks of her very much as a mother figure. When he is with her he can feel a bit of his mum in the air and he relaxes into a comfortable pattern that links him directly back to his childhood and a place of soothing nostalgia.

On a scorching summer's day on our favourite island we trundled up a dirt track that led us up a steep hill that seemed to go nowhere. How on earth could anyone live up such a treacherous hill with no signposts or street lamps? We passed several old push-bikes decorated with rust and faded by the relentless sun. This apparently was the sign that we were headed in the right direction. I already liked this place.

When we arrived at the top of the endless and seemingly corrugated hillside, Bonny's house came into view. It was built by Bonny and her husband Angel when her now grown-up children were tiny. Each brick was stacked with love and flair, each exotic-looking door panel reclaimed and lovingly restored, each knotted beam dripping with a grapevine was handpicked and laid with care. Before I could take in any more of this house that looked like a Pinterest board, out wafted Bonny. The smallest, slightest wisp of a fairy, draped in a white kaftan that made her look ethereal and almost like she was floating. Her long plaited hair seemed to travel in another time zone, catching up with her as she skipped towards us. Our first hug was like every one that has followed – strong. She hugs you like a long-lost friend and then looks in your eyes so that you feel she can read all of your secrets.

In the middle of Bonny's house is a large terrace that overlooks the ocean, all framed by a network of hanging crystals and wind chimes. There are so many other beating hearts in this home – I'm not sure how many pets reside at this hillside paradise but I certainly always feel outnumbered. This serene terrace is where Bonny and her family and friends eat freshly picked figs, the sweetest melon I've ever tasted and local creamy yogurt. This is also where we have spent some delicious moments chatting and listening to each other. Each summer I so enjoy being bathed in Bonny's energy and husky storyteller voice, all the perfect natural antidote to London life. Instant calm. Bonny has had a thousand adventures, has followed her gut and gone with the twists and turns that life has presented her with. She lives totally in the moment and without concern for how her life may differ to others. I'm constantly inspired by this wonderful friend, whether it be on balmy evenings when I'm treated to juicy tales of the 70s or over email where she'll tell me how her many pets are faring and how the quiet Ibiza winters move along with grace and serenity.

Let's hear Bonny's take on life and calm.

F: Whenever I come to your beautiful home I always feel an instant wash of calm over my body and mind. Would you say you feel calm most of the time?

B: Most of the time.

F: Have you got calmer as the years have passed by?

B: Definitely.

F: When you've been hit with unexpected adversity over the years, how have you reacted?

B: If the adversity is not of a personal nature – such as living through the experience of a major typhoon, or earthquake (done both!) or having to deal with a scarcity of income – then I have no fear! I trust implicitly that all will be well, and in the meantime, I do whatever needs to be done.

However, I totally crumble when the adversity affects my emotions – rejection and betrayal in relationships, loss of loved ones.

F: When you look back over your life from where you are now, do you think you'd react differently in those moments?

B: Looking back over my life there are obvious milestones along the way where a different choice would have led to a different outcome. But whatever the choice that was made in the moment, that was the one for that moment. At that time you don't know what you don't know.

F: How do you personally route back to calm?

B: Stop. Breathe! Feel gratitude and love for Life. Send love to all those who are suffering. Feel Love . . . Love . . . Love . . . Gratitude!

F: What is calm to you? A place? A person? A thought? A discipline?

B: Calm to me is a state of being. Simply being; floating along down the river of life. It can be felt in a place that transmits a powerful calm energy, and in the company of a person who is peaceful and centred. Calm thoughts bring calm. As a discipline it's the practice of the lessons of 'Acceptance' and 'Letting Go'.

F: What things in life throw you off balance and make you feel far from calm?

B: Arrogance, ignorance, despotism and inequality between the sexes push my buttons. There are obviously many major issues that are challenging our existence. Listing them loses the calm!

F: One of things I love about you the most is the fact that you live 100 per cent in the moment. How important do you think this is to your wellbeing?

B: Thanks to Eckhart Tolle's brilliant book, *The Power of Now*, and The Guide's teachings in The Little Guide Book, I have been learning the practice of living in the moment and this has profoundly transformed my life. When living as fully present in the moment as possible, there is a different rhythm to life. Our society has conditioned us to value who we are by what we do. There is a constant pressure to achieve. This is an insidious fear for our survival. By focusing on the present moment there is no room for fear. There is just the being. Being present. Being aware of one's part in the miracle that is Life. Living in love, harmony and gratitude.

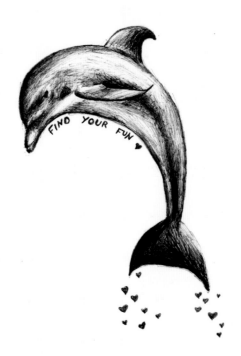

UN-CALM TYPES

So we've talked about those beloved folk who centre and calm us to the very core, but what about those who do the absolute opposite? Why did they enter our narratives in the first place? What use are they and how can we still act calmly around them? You may work with someone who makes your cheeks flush red with anger at the mere opening of their mouth. You may have a friend who has changed beyond recognition but you still feel loyal to the history of your friendship. Perhaps you're entangled in someone else's story unnecessarily and it's drowning your calm completely.

It is inevitable that we will cross paths and become caught up in the lives of others who extinguish that glorious centred feeling in one fell swoop. You may even love someone who has this effect on you, or perhaps have no love for this person, which makes this whole transaction a lot less forgivable.

I have challenging and incongruous people in my life, just like everyone else does, and even if I don't have to interact with them daily or on a deep level they still make me feel flustered and stressed – which is a one-way ticket away from my place of calm. So what is the route back and how do we get something out of it all along the way? If we are open to learning, the lessons will be there for the taking, even if they are massively annoying at first glance. If we always try to remember this, it makes the situation that bit more palatable. We also need to remember that these are all opportunities for us to fine-tune how we REACT. Why do certain people grate on us continuously and bring up bubbling chaos from the pit of our stomachs? How do they have the power to spin us around so we are disorientated and lose sight of calm altogether? Well they don't, WE choose to let them. If we bring the power back to our side of the court and remember that how we REACT is key, we can tread carefully back to the greener grass of calm.

There are many options to choose from when reacting to someone else's chaos. Fundamentally it boils down to coming at it from a place of love or fear. If it's fear, why is that our initial reaction? If we can untangle that from the other person's behaviour we have a better chance of being able to react from a more balanced place with a lot more ease. This does not mean letting others have their way, or letting them walk all over us, it simply gives us the stability and control to react calmly and put our point across firmly but from a grounded place.

Sometimes it can feel that there are 'bad guys' in our stories; menacing types who have turned up with one purpose only: to create havoc in our lives. I'm pretty sure that most of these people are actually just going about their own business without much thought at all. Some people just aren't so good at taking a look around them and seeing how their own behaviour affects others. Ignorance is much more prevalent than premeditated attacks. That individual is probably much more concerned with their own problems and fears in life, rather than their focus being annoying us.

Of course, there are some people out there who have a dark story that has led them to act in a way that does seem intentional and calculated, and I guess the only way of making sense of their actions is to look at why they ended up living life in such a way. I wish I could say the caveat to this is that 'some people are just morons', but I would be doing a disservice to myself and them to not take a closer look at the stories beneath their surface actions. Sometimes we like to diminish someone's existence to being a villainous creature who only makes bad decisions because then we can make sense of their behaviour and feel safe in our own story. We think categorising people as 'good' or 'bad' brings order to the mess that life sometimes presents. I have done this many times but I know deep down that actually everyone is struggling in their own way, which in turn leads them to act in a manner we might not agree with. We all need to drop the tags we put on people – designating them to a place of only good or evil – and see everyone as struggling humans trying to find their way.

It's actually terribly sad that some people feel they have no other option than to inflict their own pain and suffering on others. Send those people sympathy and love, as they clearly need to find another way.

Deal with those people who test your calm by taking a breath before you react, remembering where your own irritation is coming from and remembering that deep down they are probably suffering too.

A STRESS-RELIEVER

Forgiveness can be a spiky concept to embrace, too – everything about it can feel wrong in certain situations – but it can have many healing and stress-relieving qualities. Here's what I've learned about forgiveness:

Forgiveness is not about letting someone off the hook. Forgiveness doesn't necessarily dilute the wrongdoings of someone else, nor does it wipe it from history. If you have felt pain, stress or worry inflicted by another, those feelings are very real to

Forgiving others is very tricky at times as situations are loaded and some people are in your life whom you would rather were not. But forgiveness essentially frees us from them, so it's always worth it no matter how tough. Mark where you believe you are on the ripples of forgiveness and see how you could progress to the next ring in.

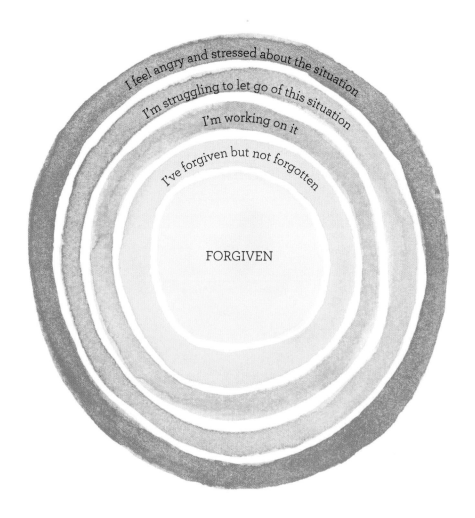

I feel angry and stressed about the situation

I'm struggling to let go of this situation

I'm working on it

I've forgiven but not forgotten

FORGIVEN

you. Forgiveness is much more about gifting yourself freedom from the shackles of the past. As soon as you properly forgive someone you can start to let go of a whole heap of stagnant stress that no longer serves you. If a friend has mistreated you, disrespected your friendship or crossed a line, you may be clinging on to a planet-sized ball of stress. This lump could be weighing you down, holding you back or creating physical problems for you. You really don't need to hold on to any of it anymore, so cut it free and forgive. If you forgive, and truly mean it, that tie can be severed quite quickly and you can be free from the past and the emotions that surround it. The longer you choose to hold on to that particular story, the longer you'll be dragged down. It might not always be easy to forgive, but if you think of it as a gift to yourself rather than to the other person involved, it can feel that bit easier.

THE SENSE OF AN ENDING

Have you ever felt so close to a friend and knew you were definitely made to be a team? A partner made for fun, adventure AND an instant route to your inner calm? Friendships like this can feel invincible, yet of course life's everchanging face can gradually change this. So what do you do when the demands of life, family and work strain your strands of history and common ground and cracks start appearing? How is it possible that a friendship that was so strong and built on similarity and connection can change gradually with life's plot twists?

It goes back to thinking of our lives as lengthy theatre productions, where characters come and go and seem to step into the spotlight at the exact moment

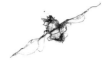

needed. I have had friendships disintegrate over time for no apparent reason. There were no disagreements or volatile scenes in our story, just time and tiny nuances moving the blocks on which our friendship was built. There isn't one specific point in time where these friendships announce their expiration; often it's a slow fizzle out without explanation. A lot less painful than a huge ruckus but it's still sad and mourned in its own way.

The next step in finding calm in this situation is to find new ways to interact with these people who were once so close and try to understand each other from our newly established vantage points. When I have encountered this sort of breakdown of understanding over the years I've been struck with worry and insecurity that it is ME who has changed and morphed into a person that is less desirable as a friend, and this has taken me far from my cosy place of calm. I am now more in the belief that everyone is permanently changing and that this either forges friendships or subtly severs ties that no longer need to be there. It's almost out of our control. We change according to what life presents us with and that may or may not match up to those around you. If you keep doing what you believe is right for you in life and what makes you happy and calm, those who are like-minded will be attracted into the picture. Those people who don't may not work harmoniously with how you see life, and that is fine, too. I believe we attract the right people at the right time, even if it feels strange, uncomfortable and sometimes very tough.

It's almost as if we are all marbles, rolling around all corners of the earth, bashing into other marbles that ping us off into different directions. If we remember that new routes may lead us to personal expansion then whatever happens to our friendships we can continue to be in that calm place. Keep rolling, keep moving and know you're going to bump into some seriously brilliant marbles along the way.

STEER AWAY FROM OVERANALYSING

I often find myself bubbling with panic about things I've said to friends and acquaintances. This makes me lose my grounded footing as I start sprinting in the opposite direction of calm. In fact, I can't even imagine calm when I'm in this state as everything seems magnified and too vivid to focus on the stable things in life. I've wasted hours, days, weeks worrying about exchanges I've had with friends or new acquaintances, wishing I could turn back the clock and start over again. I'm sure most of these occurrences were disposed of quite instantly by the others involved but for me they usually play on loop, tormenting me over and over again.

I speak for a living and get a lot out of general communication. I adore how ideas can spring from seemingly dry wells and sparks of magic appear when words are exchanged; it sets me on fire and makes me feel excited about life. The flip side to this is 'expectation'. I always want that human connection to feel at ease, positive and flowing. The anticipation of these wants when I meet someone new can get me wrapped in nerves which dilute my usual ability to say what I'm truly feeling. I start to second guess what others want me to say and then lose my natural flow of honest communication. I hate it when this happens as I get tangled in knots of insecurity and fear. I suffer angst that they won't like me, will judge me too quickly or make me feel rejected. It seems much easier to be perked up by others' love and kind words than to dig deep and find that self-acceptance alone. When I have these post-conversation panics I try to look back to remembering that as long as I was honest and just being me, the rest is irrelevant.

I have learned over the years to take my fair share of responsibility for the outcome of life around me. At times I take this on board a little too much and completely eradicate anyone else in the situation. When friendships have broken down, wires have been crossed and disagreement flares up, I tend to carry the full weight of the outcome without recalling that there was another involved. I recently opened up to a friend about this guilt and she suggested looking at it in a different way to see if that took the sharp edge off. First, she asked if perhaps my regretful actions could have acted as a catalyst for others to take a closer look in the mirror, to recognise things they needed to change in their own lives. I had never given this a thought and could see some truth in it.

My friend then went on to wonder whether in these moments I acted a certain way because I was locking into the chaotic orbit and discomfort of others. I could see specks of truth in this, too. This doesn't allow me to extract myself from the outcome of these transactions and get away scot-free, but it certainly allows me to look at certain portions of my history from a calmer place. I'm not dodging my own bullet of responsibility, but I feel a little lighter and much calmer about it now that I've looked at it from many angles (and this is another good example of why a friend's perspective can be a godsend).

What I've learned from these moments is to 'let it go'. Know that, yes, you could have said something more genuine, funnier, smarter, cooler, gentler, but the moment has passed, no intentional damage was implied and you have learned from it. Send that anxiety sailing off into the sunset, as once you've learned your lesson it simply does not serve you anymore. We must not let these moments define us or swallow us up.

If you are really suffering from overanalysing a past situation, you could try one of a few more tangible tricks that I've tried over the years that I find really soothing and most definitely take me back to a place of calm. One is to write letters. Think of that friend or acquaintance and what you feel discomfort about and put down those words in ink that you have never said out loud. Say sorry, say that you wished you had played things differently, say you forgive them, say you felt hurt, say that you are ready to free yourself of these heavy shackles, and then burn the letter and watch that moment fracture and drift into the air. After a while, and certainly after we've learned those lessons, that baggage just becomes an uncomfortable mass blocking our view of calm. It blindsides us and muffles our ears from the sounds nearby. We don't have to carry those regrets and that torment around for life.

Another way of doing this is to imagine that person in front of you. Go to a calm and quiet place in your home and picture them sitting there looking at you. Speak to them openly and honestly and let the words roll, unrehearsed and naturally. Release those words out of your mouth and into the air to be carried away far from where you sit. You don't need those words and worries trapped inside you anymore, so release them into the wild along with the anxiety they harbour. It doesn't matter how or where you do these little ceremonies but it will count and make you feel much lighter. If you are feeling strong and centred you could even try sending a letter or speaking to the person in question. You could tell them how you really feel and that you have regret and remorse about how you acted and perhaps question their actions too. Say whatever feels comfortable and alleviating to you!

DON'T LET PEOPLE
TAKE THE PISS

Some of us will be people pleasers, some of us will be piss takers, some of us will be shy and retiring, and others loud and proud. Where do you sit in it all and can you clearly see the role you play in those around you?

Dealing with people who take a mile when offered an inch can be tricky, and it's a lesson I've learned many times over. I think I am a fair person generally and I also love to give. I get a huge kick out of lending my time, energy and resources to those I love in life, as I believe that transaction is hugely important. This has been abused over the years at times, and it seems to be something I am still trying to manage. What leaps out is that I'm not very good at setting boundaries. Setting boundaries means I can still freely give and offer up my time and energy but I do have my limits before it all starts to affect me.

Over the years a few acquaintances have taken a giant leap over that line of decency, which I always find shocking as I would not personally feel comfortable doing the same. Again, this acts as a huge reminder that I should always be clear with

Sometimes it is easy to believe that our past mistakes or history define us. It's time to truly remember that we can write our own story. If there are some memories or a person who you feel takes over your head, write it down here and realise it doesn't define you – it's a story that you can rewrite.

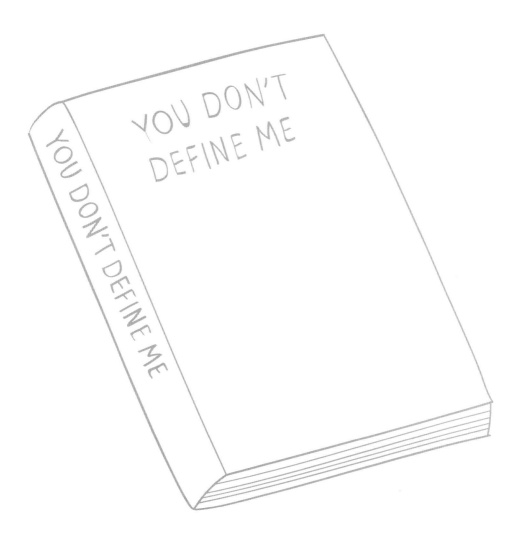

my outlines in these moments. If someone in your life continually decides to cross the line and takes advantage of whatever you're offering, be brave and communicate that they no longer have that access to your time or energy.

PEER PRESSURE

I don't believe that friendship has to rest on the foundations of similarity. It doesn't have to be bound together by convenient geography, synchronised ages or paralleled backgrounds. Any important friendship in your life will invariably stand out because of a connection. An inexplicable magic that brings out the best in both of you and opens your mind to new possibilities.

As much as we adore our friends we don't have to think exactly like them to all get along and journey through life together. As the years roll on I have oscillated between sticking to this idea and butting my head against it. At times I am inspired by friends and their actions, and their motivation has given me that get up and go that I needed. Some wonderful friends have achieved personal goals, shown huge amounts of courage or stood up for what they believe and this has led to me focus on their determination and try to emulate it in my own way. This is one of the great hidden dimensions of friendship. We egg each other on without truly realising it. We inspire each other, push each other and remind each other of our full potential.

The flip side to this is going against the grain. Just because the masses are headed in one direction doesn't mean that we have to follow suit. Even if our friends' actions are widely celebrated, proven to work or simply the 'norm', it doesn't mean we have to stay with the flock. I love going against the grain but it has taken years and lots of enforced confidence to get me to the place where I know how to follow my own instinct.

A small example of this would be how I like to live my life at present. My life is split into only a few portions. The main one is family life. Spending time with my husband, kids and step-kids and making sure that the family machine runs well and smoothly. The next segment is work. I love my many jobs and their creative flow; each project reignites a passion and flame within which makes me feel 100 per cent alive. Then comes friends and down time. This to me means yoga, the odd calm lunch meet-up with friends, painting, reading and getting into the great outdoors. In my twenties I used to love nothing more than sinking a strong gin and tonic at a noisy bar, but those times have slipped away for now. They may come back, but that need to get intoxicated and alter my own mental state has left the building in this period of my life. Time seems too precious and busy to add getting drunk regularly and encouraging chaos into the mix. Some of my friends have accepted this new flow of life without question, whereas others see my new choices as boring. This is fine by me, as I know I'm making the right choices for me at this point in my life. I want to have energy for my children and creativity, so going out regularly for nighttime adventures doesn't fit into the mix.

There is no right or wrong but what needs to be respected are people's choices. Some of our friends will always have a wild streak. Some will have a family, some might not. Some will spend the majority of their time and energy on things we don't see the

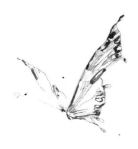

point of, and more than likely vice versa. We are all different and have varying routes to take for hundreds of contrasting reasons. This is what makes friendship fun.

We must all keep our cool when our friendship circle has different ideas to us. Don't get the fear of missing out, there is no point. You made a decision to go about things in YOUR way so honour that and enjoy every minute if you can. Fear of missing out takes you straight out of that sweet spot of calm as you instantly feel like you might be doing something wrong. Why would YOU be the only one out there not doing what everyone else is doing? Because you chose not to somewhere down the line. You will gain what you need out of your own situation and your friends will grab hold of what they desire in theirs. Ultimately, being true to yourself will lead you to that calm place. Always remember it's okay to go against the grain. It's actually one of the most liberating paths to take.

Summary

LISTEN.

Sometimes that outside perspective is just what you need.

BE THERE.

Even when your friends aren't listening, be there for them.

GO YOUR OWN WAY.

Don't do anything just because they are – calm and happiness are personal quests.

WHAT DOES A CALM FRIENDSHIP LOOK LIKE TO YOU?

Write one word or draw a picture here that sums it up.

CALM
WORK

Some of you will read the title of this chapter and instantly shudder, whilst
others of you will beam with joy. Work can be the most divisive subject to
touch on and can sometimes be tricky terrain to navigate. I feel completely
jackpot lucky that I love my job. I found out what made me tick in the
creative department very early on in life and went full throttle into it as I
was brought up by two hardworking parents. This combination, with some
magic luck thrown in, has allowed me to have a career that has so far lasted
20 years. I can't quite believe it myself as I have never had a plan or major
fantasy, I have just kept ploughing on, going with what feels right
in my gut. Many tried to discourage me and saw my hopes as sheer
fantasy but luckily I was naive/determined enough to carry on
regardless and have had many adventures along the way.

WORK STRESS

Although I work in a field from which I get a lot of satisfaction and pleasure, it doesn't mean that my working life has been without stress. There have been mountains of it. Sometimes that mountain has been so high and treacherous to climb that I've lost my footing and stumbled backwards, wondering if I should abort the ascent altogether. There have been many moments where I have wanted to give up and throw away all my previous hard work. The reasons for this reaction are always rooted in stress.

Now I'm fully aware that I'm a showbiz wally who doesn't have to dig holes, like my wonderful hardworking dad does, all day. I don't have to deal with life-or-death matters, or carry the responsibility of a whole team. Yet my stress at work has come in strange shapes and sizes and has at times felt like it was suffocating me. My personal list of work stresses might not completely resonate with you, but I'm sure there will be similarities and links that you can relate to no matter what job you have chosen to do in life. But first let me take you back to where it all started.

MY OWN WORK STRESSES

I'm 15 and sat in a felt-floored waiting area with 50 or so other girls my age. They all look much more outgoing and confident than me and are much prettier. They are without puppy fat and are wearing seemingly much more sophisticated outfits. I was quite proud of my Wembley Market PVC trench coat and cord slacks until I entered this room of mini Britney Spears lookalikes. I had been to several auditions prior to this one but felt out of my depth as I knew nothing about presenting, which is what this role was about. It's safe to say that I 100 per cent blagged every inch of the audition. This was probably because I didn't feel too much stress in these situations when I was younger, as I had an eternal optimism that came from lack of experience in the 'loss and lessons' department. I felt the nerves, for sure, but my awareness of outside judgment was minuscule in comparison to what it became later down the line.

Getting my first job on *The Disney Club* was one of the best moments of my career. Sheer joy with no strings attached. I had been accepted into the elusive TV club and didn't care what that meant as long as I could keep my foot in the sequin-covered door. I managed to keep my head down and trundle through this strange new life whilst still doing my GCSEs, then I jumped from this kids' TV show to a few others along the way. I wasn't the best at the audition that day, but I gave it my all and went with what felt right at the time. I have tried to stick to this loose theory somewhat over the years and always try to route back to it if I feel knocked from my flow: all you can do is your best that day.

The stress came later down the line. I think a lethal concoction of entering the arena of being in the press and the initiation of social media gave my beloved job a newfound edge that I wasn't sure how to handle. To be honest, I still don't. At that point in my career, when I was steadily working but still too young to embrace who I truly was, I felt not quite good enough. I was ripped from my place of calm and compared to every other girl on TV. I was asked to dress differently by one producer who had picked up on my natural sway towards masculine clothing. I was asked to talk in a slightly softer tone by another. I was told I wasn't good enough by tonnes of them.

This is when I started to look at the girl from the north-west London suburbs in tomboy clothes and pick holes at her in every way possible. This newly opened pothole stopped me seeing any good in myself, as nobody else seemed to. If I didn't get a job I was up for I felt worthless. As the power of the internet grew, if someone was mean about me online I felt a hole widening in the pit of my stomach. A new empty cavity reserved for self-loathing and hate. The whole of my self-esteem hung in the hands of others – I had no grasp of self-belief or identity without their validation. At times like this calm was a very far-off place. I had at a very young age been openly judged, objectified and tossed to one side so many times and I didn't know how to process what was really going on.

THE REALITY OF FAME

When ver I hear youngsters say they would like to be famous my toes curl up inside my shoes. What does fame even mean these days? It certainly doesn't entail the glossy Hollywood shimmer of yesteryear. There is little sacred mystery or fantasy about it these days at all. We know everything, or at least think we do. Now let's get a few things straight before I continue this much-needed rant. Firstly I know I'm not Beyoncé and can quite happily walk down my local high street with very little bother. Secondly I know that there are far more important issues to rant upon but I still think for the concern of a portion of the younger generation growing up and exposed to so much, it's worth a mini rant. Thirdly I am highly aware of the fact that I have hosted shows that promote pointless fame earlier on in my career. I'm not responsible for those contestants wanting it or thinking they wanted it and I actually had a lot of fun on these shows along the way. Lessons are learned and people change. So onwards . . . I didn't get into TV to be famous. I had no concept of what it was beyond knowing that all my friends and I were in love with this chap called Leonardo DiCaprio with complete knowledge we would never meet him. I got in to TV because I loved everything about it. The buzz, the energy, the excitement, the possible travel, the new people. I wanted in because of that. The fame came gradually and steadily and I've had 20 years to get used to the idea but I do need to break some myths that surround it to make my point. Being famous does not mean you are free of worry, pain or stress. It doesn't offer up the glowing feeling of achievement as the two are unrelated. It doesn't mean you feel better about yourself or more whole as a human and it doesn't offer up any glamour, even if, at times, it lead to exciting people and places. I'll now tell you exactly how fame feels to me. Imagine you are walking down a quite dirt track enjoying the sunshine and the pleasant view. There is a barb wire fence to your left that you haven't really noticed as you take in the fresh air and colours around you. All of a sudden you are awoken from your peaceful state by a loud and sudden barking. You look to your left and there are 20 dogs all on hind legs, paws hooked into the mesh of the fence, mouths wide, barking their heads off at you. You know they cant get you or physically hurt you in anyway but it's disturbing and unnervin. A constant stare, judgment and often attacked for the wrong reason or misinformed opinion.

These days this side of my job still causes me certain amounts of stress but I try to pay less attention to it. I can't say I'm completely immune to the side-effects of this sort of exposure but I'm certainly content enough in myself to know that I'm okay without the constant approval of others. I'm not saying this for sympathy, I'm just trying to shed light on what it's really all about. Fame isn't something I think about at all day-to-day. It's not until I'm alerted to outside judgment or abuse that I take any notice at all.

STRESS POINTS

Another element of my job that I still cannot find the calm in is being interviewed. I really struggle with it. Before the journalist has even opened their notepad I feel the sweats coming on. Again, I am fully aware that this is not a life-or-death situation and I really should be saving the 'fight-or-flight' mode for something far more important but I feel spooked by the whole situation. Some of the journalists I have been interviewed by have been lovely and written fair and observational pieces about me, but the few who have grilled me and twisted my words have left me with a sour taste in my mouth that I can't quite wash away. I am on high alert and know that every word I say, every move I make is being duly noted and assessed. Assumptions are made and calculations worked out from tiny snippets of information seen with a single set of eyes. I sink back to being a 13-year-old at school not knowing how to spell a certain word as these invariably well-educated people sit and quiz me to suss out if I'm 'good enough'. I know that's not what they're actually doing but my own personal bad habit is to slip into this way of thinking. I take full responsibility for that one. However, I'm terrified that my words will morph and have new meaning by the time they reach the Dictaphone and that my true stories and ideas will be instead steeped in judgment by the time they hit the printed page. I'm not sure I have ever felt calm in an interview, but hey, that's another challenge to quietly work on.

No matter what job we do, I think there will always be weak spots that take us away from calm, even if you love what you do. There are parts of my career that I fall into with ease and a carefree air that allows me to be my best. When I'm writing I feel so happy and content and very little stress shows at all. I know I'm not the best writer out there but my veins buzz with pumping blood when I get a good flow going. Unbeatable. When I'm on the radio I feel accepted and welcome and I love the rapport I get from the listeners. I really enjoy the fun side of social media and how that allows me to talk to and hear the ideas of many people who are engaging in what I do. These feel like spaces where I am confident and in control to some extent.

When I'm on TV I don't always have that luxury. It might be something to do with being seen AND heard that feels so massively exposing, unlike in the comfort of my radio chair where I can hide behind a giant mic and beautiful songs. I am also acutely aware of how amazing so many other broadcasters are and how at ease they seem in front of the camera. Although I've worked in TV for 20 years, at times I still feel off centre when the cameras go on. This feeling leaves me when the first few minutes have passed and I've got into my groove, but initially I lose my calm.

SOME CONFIDENCE TRICKS

I know a lot of other people in the business who get stage fright, even the more seasoned performers. I've had many discussions on how to harness this unnerving energy and put it to use in a positive way, and these tricks help you to gather this energy and give it permission to propel you dynamically rather than leaving you static in the headlights, which might mean you find you're more alert and that bit sharper when you really need to be.

These are all tricks that can be used in most professions, not just the entertainment industry. If you have to speak in front of colleagues at work you may have experienced the same heart-pounding sensation. Speaking in public may feel vastly unnatural to you and in those moments it's near impossible to feel calm. One thing I always try to remember is that the room you're talking to isn't occupied with people all waiting for you to slip up. More than likely, they're willing you along or hoping to gain something from what you say. If we eradicate the possibility of everyone wanting us to fail we stand a good chance of getting back in the driving seat with confidence and calm. It's much like that classic line: 'imagine the audience naked' which brings this sentiment back to its bare bones. We are all human; we all have the same body parts under those distracting garments, and we all most definitely make mistakes. Those who judge freely and without thought are not recognising their own mishaps and mistakes in life but are living a very closed and narrow existence. Remember this fact if you have to speak in front of others or in moments where you feel judged for your efforts. It's a good one for job interviews, too!

Slowing everything down a notch is also a good trick when you feel the nerves creeping into those previously calm spaces. Adrenaline and fear ramp us up to our highest speed where mistakes are more prevalent and breath escapes us. If you slow down your movements and words your pumping heart will hopefully follow suit, you'll sound more in control and more confident in your approach. Take time to concentrate on the words you are pronouncing and keep your breaths long and steady. This is my focus at work – often!

DETERMINING PRIORITIES

When I had my first-born, Rex, my perspective changed greatly and my stresses altered along with my new way of thinking. I had less time to worry about what others thought of my choices and mishaps at work but the way in which I managed my time now seemed to me to be of paramount importance. Finding this balance in life still makes my face heat up and my muscles tense. I don't want to let my kids down and I don't want to fail at work. This constant balancing act often makes me feel like a failure in every department, which I know is a feeling that many parents share. After having Rex I knew I needed to make some changes to ease the juggling act a little, and it wasn't easy. I still struggle with this one to this day, but I did have a bit of an epiphany recently.

Whilst writing this book I've been taking a much more detailed inventory of how I deal with stress and the reasons why I lose my calm. As I closed my laptop after completing the first full draft of this book, another lesson was waiting to unfold. I figured that by this point I had written down most of my thoughts on the subject and had looked in depth at my own perception of stress and calm, but this particular weekend opened up a whole new channel of thought.

My husband was away on a work trip and I was looking after the four kids on my own. I love it when our house is full and I adore watching my kids and step-kids all merge as a frenetic yet harmonious unit. The joy I feel when the house is reverberating with noise and love is divine, yet it is equalled by an overwhelming expectation of chaos. It is inevitable; there will be multiple meals cooked, mountains of washing, several disagreements, varying movements and a lot of cleaning (even in the madness I have to keep my sideboards sparkling, I can't help it!) and amongst all this I will be trying to keep my career ticking over. In this moment of anticipation, it dawned on me that when I lose my calm, nine times out of 10 it'll be because I'm trying to fight the chaos. I'll be searching for remedies to lessen the chaos, trying to fire-fight the mess and debris of family life, or trying to make sense of the general anarchy that is created when five people are in the house with very different agendas. This impossible feat, at times, drives me mad. I will start the day in battle mode, ready to quash any sofa stain or lack-of-toy-sharing with my emphatic need to control it all. But I've realised that the movements of these four wonderful people in my life will not change. There is no chance of their social wants, dietary needs or spontaneous thoughts aligning, so it is up to me to change my perception of it all.

EMBRACE THE CHAOS

This is where I stumbled across the glaringly obvious thought that I must 'EMBRACE THE CHOAS'. I have to lay down my surface spray and other chaos-battling weapons and accept everything that comes with the kids. Maybe I could even learn to enjoy it? Not just the mess but the fizzing energy that swarms a house when it's full to the brim with individuals. This energy previously had the potential to make me feel very overwhelmed and as if I had no time for myself. Maybe in practical terms this is true, but what if I could find those moments amongst the madness? What if I could recognise what I was getting back for me in the transaction of being part of this frenzied family life? All the joy, love, learning and entertainment of having such a wonderfully big and beautifully chaotic family.

So I gave it a try. My husband's return flight got delayed by a day so I had even more time to practise this one and feel the rewards. With my new mental approach, the stress was diluted, the busyness felt manageable and I enjoyed almost all of it. Rather than adopting my usual tactic of trying to build a raft to skim over choppy water, I took a dive straight in. It is SO much less exhausting and therefore much easier to route back to calm as you're not desperately scrambling for it in the first place.

My go-to tactic when everything feels chaotic while I'm trying to juggle work and family is to fire-fight it, but now I'm trying to accept it and am getting closer to calm in these situations. We may all be searching desperately for some calm, but perhaps we have to learn how to accept chaos fully first?

WORK-LIFE BALANCE

Making big changes in your working life – even if you know you need to for your wellbeing's sake – can be excruciating as there are so many factors to take into account. If you love your job you'll be worried about reducing your hours or switching things up in case you don't get to do it anymore. If you hate your job but desperately want change you'll be worried about how you will get food on the table and pay the bills without it. Sometimes you'll be bound by habit. As a hangover to my old work patterns, if I see a week in my work diary with not much planned I feel like my career is slipping away from me. PANIC!

At times you can feel trapped and oppressed by the lack of options that lie ahead. If you can't leave your job or switch things up right now is there someone at your workplace you can talk to who might just understand how you're feeling? Is there a hobby or form of creative escape you can counterbalance your work life with in your free time? Quite a few of my mates now have jobs on the side which don't feel like work at all. They're hobbies that offer up light relief from their full-time jobs but also a little income. One friend has a home decor blog online, one runs a clothes-customising business from her home and one is learning to be a yoga teacher. Sometimes it might even help just to apply for new jobs or scout around for them even if it doesn't feel like a realistic move right now. Put those ideas and thoughts out there to test the water and see how differing opportunities make you feel.

How balanced do you believe your life is? Do you work way too much and let the rest of your life suffer? Do you let stress in because of this? Do you shy away from work because you have fears of failing or are just simply not sure what you want out of it all? Write down what you believe takes up most of your time in the heavier scale and put all other activities in the other. Then look at how you might be able to balance them out.

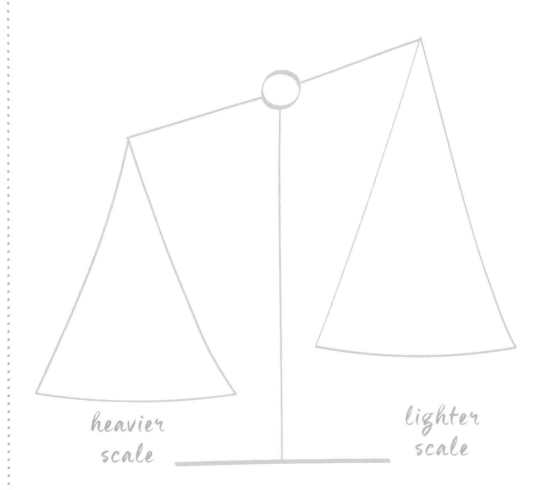

heavier
scale

lighter
scale

ANYTHING IS POSSIBLE

This is a great story for anyone who wants to make a big change and needs some confidence to take the gamble. One of my great friends, Justine Jenkins, was working in the City for the majority of her twenties. She worked hard, doing long hours bustling in the craziness of the banking world with little time off and a constant need to keep up with the velocity of the City. Deep down she always craved something different but didn't know where to start. Her true passion was make-up and creativity, which seemed worlds away from her current place in numbers and high-octane stress. She had no training or experience in the make-up world so at first thought she would make it a hobby. She managed to persuade a local theatre to let her come and do work experience in her free time. Due to the long hours in a fired-up office she would have to tag this time onto the end of long days or at weekends, but through dedication and sheer drive she made this hobby gain momentum by talking to people in the industry and by getting more experience, which in turn led to a surge of confidence. She knew that leaving the City would mean very little income for an unknown quantity of time, but she thought it was worth the sacrifice. She had managed to save a little to get by and finally hung up her 80s power suit along with a whole heap of stress. The next chapter of her life was a slog but a beautiful one. It was low pay, non-existent security, yet pure joy. She loved every minute of this creative process and due to the time and energy she invested into her new vocation, she started to feel like she was getting somewhere. She soon found herself on several sets of big movies and TV shows, working alongside many people she had previously admired from afar. Her pay still didn't match her City salary but the pay off in regards to life balance and stress was priceless. She now works constantly in editorial publication and TV and has a constant supply of work and loyal fans. It was all a huge gamble with no crashmat to land on if it all went wrong but she went with her gut feeling and followed what her heart was telling her.

I made one almighty change to my own life when I left Radio 1. As much as I loved the job and felt honoured to hold the title, I felt there was more to explore out there and other ways to experience creative flow. I had had the most brilliant adventure interviewing so many astounding artists and had witnessed live world-class music. The mere thought of leaving felt ludicrous but I had this itch; this tiny scratch that turned into an omnipresent dig, telling me to switch things up. I knew the pressure of not making a single mistake whilst talking for three hours a day had taken its toll along the way and that I also needed some quiet time away from my own dialogue and fear of slipping up in public. I knew it was a gamble as I had a small child in tow and no fall-back at all. No one would be able to scrape me out of this mess if it all fell to pieces. Still, I followed my gut and spoke those seminal words aloud. 'I'm going to leave.' This tiny sentence was met with every imaginable response. 'YOU ARE MAD!' 'Why would you leave a secure job like that?' 'What if you never work again?' 'You might lose your place within the music industry forever.' Each time I felt bombarded with terror. I couldn't grasp that initially calm thought that had entered my head randomly one day the first time I made the decision to go. At the time, the decision for change felt expansive and grounded rather than wild and crazy, but all of these responses were making me lose my confidence in it completely.

Having dreams isn't foolish or unrealistic. We all deserve to have dreams and to believe in them. This doesn't mean we can expect them to happen quickly or even as we imagined but hey . . . anything is possible! Once you have a clear goal of what your dream is, it can be a lot of fun walking that bit closer to it. Write down your main work goal or dream at the top of the steps, then write down a few things you believe could lead you in the right direction on the steps climbing up to it.

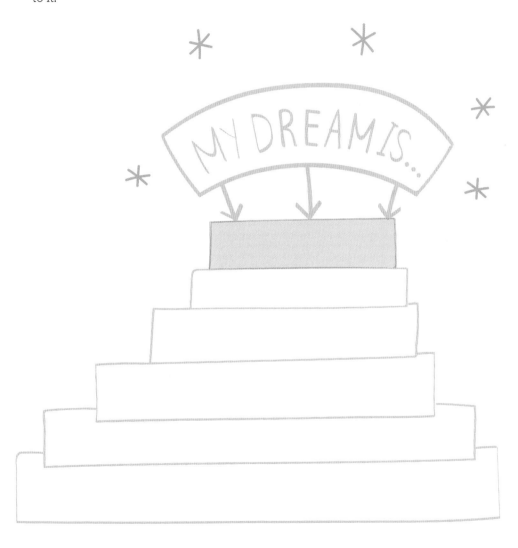

The first six months after my departure were freeing yet simultaneously wretched. I saw the future as a blank page, which on a good day was enthralling and tantalising, but on a bad day was full of doom and gloom. The unknown could show up as a delightful friend with tonnes of ideas, or a shadowy character void of opportunity. This is the gamble you take when making big changes, but how you process that worry and how you drive on through it counts more than ever. I learned how important it is to stay positive and believe in yourself, and that leaps of faith can lead you to new fun places.

I found calm during those first months by doing what I loved – being creative. I kept writing even if nobody read my words, I kept painting even if my paintings never left my kitchen and I kept talking about ideas and dreams as if hey would 100 per cent come to fruition. This was a great breeding ground for positivity to grow.

I look back at that period now with a sense of relief because I'm currently working on various projects that make my skin tingle with excitement when I think about them. It might not be everyone's cup of tea, but for me writing and creating is where my heart is at. For some of you it'll be numbers and working out problems. It could be physical and outdoors. Looking after children or teaching. Even if you haven't worked out what makes you tick there will most definitely be something out there that will feel right to you at some point. It doesn't matter about the title of the job or its size; it's what it brings to you that matters. When people ask me what I do for a living now, I have no answer. I don't have a title or set of accolades that box me into a single category, and that's fine by me. For me that IS calm. It's not about titles or power or accolades, it's about pure enjoyment. Do you feel it's possible to find your calm at work, if not now then later down the line? Perhaps from change, or seeking out what you truly love and adding it to the side of what you already do? Our own visions of calm at work will differ massively, so listen to your heart and the answer will be there.

BE HONEST

There have, of course, been times when I have not loved all the jobs I've worked on. There are shows that I decided to be part of that didn't ever feel quite right. I took the opportunity out of fear that I would fall behind others and felt they were the sort of jobs I SHOULD be doing. This to me is the opposite of calm.

I also worked with people who I didn't see eye to eye with, and struggled with the chaos that this sort of transaction delivers. If your boss is a bully or one of your colleagues makes things tricky at work it can feel impossible to stay true to what you believe is right. I am not the best at confrontation at work as I find the words get stuck in my throat and my neck burns like a firework about to go off. At times I have a tendency to people-please and therefore compromise my own beliefs to avoid difficult moments. This is always a bad idea. Being honest with those around you, even if it means having that toe-curling chat, is always a better option than storing up resentment and stress.

I once worked with a colleague who I didn't always see eye to eye with. I'm sure they felt the same about me as we had very different ideas and outlooks on many work-related subjects. I was much younger so I felt I didn't have the clout to oppose the decisions that were being made on my behalf. The words and differences of opinion I so desperately wanted to express would dissolve within seconds of walking in the door at work. Instead I felt frustration towards this person and our relationship became stilted. In fairness, we were both going about the situation in the wrong way; without compromise or movement. This does not make for a calm work environment at all.

These days I have got better at saying my piece. This doesn't mean I have to be mean or unnecessarily outspoken, it just means I'm honest and authentic with my words and actions. I find that this helps to dissolve the stress that bit quicker. If I speak honestly, as hard as this might be, I can let go of the stress that would more than likely turn into resentment. I think this is a lesson we learn with time and experience. It's taken me almost 20 years to get to the place where I feel I can flex these muscles but what I've learned is that it removes so much stress from the situation. Your honest words may be met with shock or even anger but those reactions will most definitely dissipate after your colleague has digested them and taken them on board with a level of respect.

On top of that, your work mates or boss may be instantly impressed and taken aback by your honesty, which could lead to bridging new relationships and fresh ways of working. If you're honest it's all up for grabs! We must always remember that those around us who seem powerful and strong are no different to us. They started out at a similar level to us and once had bosses and more overbearing colleagues than them. No one needs to be mean or cool to get to the places they want to reach. You can be grounded and calm and reach your own goals just as easily. Actually, more easily – as the ripple effects of your own goodwill can only be embraced and drawn in by those around you. That makes for a very calm workplace.

Even if you love your job, there is probably room for some improvements. And when you hate your job, there is ALWAYS room to make improvements. What do you feel you get out of your work at the moment and what would you like more of?

Tea

HELLO TO WOO...

In my twenties I spent a lot of time flitting between my home town of London and Los Angeles, where I was working on several projects as well as juggling my career at home. It was a whirlwind period of my life that I look back on so fondly. Adventure was rife and spontaneity led me to meet some brilliant people who have become friends for life. One of these individuals is Dr Woo, the legendary tattoo artist, whose waiting list is near impossible to get on and whose style is lusted after the world over.

When we met on a hot and bustling LA night in a crowded bar, Woo was just starting out in his tattoo career by helping with odd jobs in Shamrock Social Club, a well-known and loved tattoo shop on Sunset Boulevard. He had little experience but a lot of drive and passion.

He was taken under the wing by the king of tattoos, Mr Mark Mahoney, whose skill and individual technique precedes him. Mark has done several of my tattoos, adorning my skin with his light touch that almost looks like a pencil sketch. Mark is one of those intoxicating characters who inspires those around him and tells tales of the underground LA scene without giving away too much of his own story. Mystery and magic fill the air when he is around. He looks like a 1950s gangster but has the gentle demeanour of a friendly cartoon pirate. He saw potential and determination in Woo and gave him the time and space to develop as an artist and great talent in his own right.

Over the years Woo worked relentlessly, learning his trade. He worked as Mark's apprentice and right-hand man, tattooing the glitterati of the LA scene, always watching and always learning.

Due to his disciplined energy and focus he has become one of the most in-demand tattoo artists of our time. He has worked on nearly every recognisable inked person out there and has developed a unique style so that people can always spot a 'Dr Woo'. His creativity and skill have enabled his work to travel across the planet and for his coveted tattoos to be called pieces of art.

I have been back to LA many times over the years to reconnect with Woo and am always in awe of how he has handled this incredible rise to fame. He has stepped calmly into this new territory, remaining solidly grounded and a family man. We both started our careers at similar times and I think we both have the same outlook on work and life and the importance of balancing it all. He is a classic example of someone who has risen to the top without drama or fuss, proving you can achieve success and a lot of love without pushing and shoving your way there. I thought Woo would be the perfect person to chat to about success, determination and keeping calm throughout it all.

F: Hey Woo, I've known you for over a decade now and have so enjoyed watching you soar in your career. When we first met you were working at Shamrock Social Club with a beginner's experience but big dreams. Did you always believe you would be the best and so in demand when you were starting out?

W: Though I never actually thought I'd be where I am now and in my current situation . . . I always knew I would do my best and work hard no matter what, and this would lead me to do something great, no matter what it was. It was always a mantra I had and now I feel blessed to see it come to fruition.

F: You have always been very focused and dedicated, do you think that's what has allowed you to gain such popularity and status in the tattoo community?

W: To be honest, I think it was a bit of good timing with the rise of social media, the sincerity of my work and the reinterpretation of tattoo works we are familiar with. The aesthetic drew interest, and the digital realm spread the work.

F: When you started to succeed how did those around you react? Were any friends wary of your success? Did anyone start to treat you differently?

W: All my close friends and family were so supportive and energised. They were happy to see positive things shifting into place for me and I was always grateful. But as with all things, some people resent it and that's fine... I get it. But for the most part everyone has been great.

F: Although you are at the top of your game you seem to have remained particularly calm throughout your journey to the top. You have never come across as pushy or desperate to succeed, it's all been done with an air of calm. Is that the reality?

W: I think I'd like to believe it is! But sometimes it's not even the push to succeed or a constant effort to get to the top, it's just simply the effort to make the best of my work and be happy with myself. At the end of the day, if those things make me happy and my family is in a good place, then I'm okay with that . . . the subsequent great opportunities that come, are to me, maybe a lasting impression of that work and the rewards that come from that.

F: How do you stay calm at work when the pressure is on?

W: It's the only situation where I feel calm. I have discovered it is a very relaxing mindset for me in the chair.

F: In this day and age I believe many get sucked into believing success relies purely on status and money rather than how much you enjoy your work. What does success mean to you personally?

W: It's true, and I feel it sometimes . . . it's tough, especially in a city like LA. But before I get too caught up I always remember, true success for me is my family and their happiness . . . as long as that is right, nothing else matters.

F: Have your goals formed organically over the years or have you had a set plan?

W: To be honest, a bit of both. Pretty much I have been trying to manoeuvre the planned and unplanned events in my career and hope they work together seamlessly.

F: What else do you want to achieve in the future?

W: I have so many ideas and creative projects that I still want to get out there, and just grow this brand organically and correctly as much as I can.

"

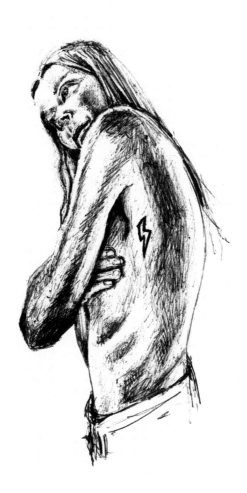

CALM, FULFILLED, SUCCESSFUL

Some people feed off stress at work and this can be massively counterproductive in so many ways. It can be very addictive, too, as you start to believe that it's the only way to get things done. In my twenties I was insanely busy as I knew no other way. I would wrap on one filming project only to jump in a cab to whiz to another that would go on until late in the evening. I would then be up at the crack of dawn to start work on something new, and so on. A complete non-stop Ferris wheel of self-imposed chasing of the ticking clock. I felt imbalanced and very chaotic, but I fed off this. I wanted more rapidity and more chaos, as the adrenaline that came as part of the package made me accelerate even more. I saw no harm in living in this way – until I crashed and burned later down the line. During this crazy and exciting period I also forgot to see what was really going on around me. The world seemed to be moving at such speed, whereas in fact it was just my head that was running at 100 mph. If you know you work in this way and feel your working life will crumble if you don't have that slight chaos to feed off, fear not. I don't allow myself to push through life at this pace any more but I am still enjoying most jobs I take on, and with the same amount of passion and drive that I always had. You don't need stress to be fulfilled or successful.

I have learned to take on slightly less but also concentrate more fully in each moment. It has been a wonderful realisation that passion doesn't have to derive from stress or pressure. Previously life was too fast to stop and smell the roses, whereas now I allow myself that bit more time to find calm. Even if your job seems steeped in chaos there will be tiny chinks of light to grab hold of to give you that much-needed

When we feel stressed at work there is often a way to help dilute these feelings if we stop and think outside of the box. Write down below what you feel most stressed about, then look at the list to see if any of these options can help with what you're dealing with.

....

....

....

....

....

....

....

Can you ask for help from another?

Can you take time for yourself in your day? Perhaps a walk to work, walk at lunchtime or stroll home afterwards.

Can you slow down and not worry about how fast everyone else is working?

Can you switch off fully when you get home and not mention work to those you live with?

Can you work out who is applying the most pressure to you? Is it your boss, your colleagues or you? Can you talk to them about it?

breather. Is it possible for you to take a step outside to breathe in fresh air? Is there an opportunity for you to shut your laptop down a little earlier than usual? Is there a way in which you can set yourself goals of how much you'll enjoy your job rather than how high you can climb?

What does success mean to you? Is it instantly related to power, or money or being better than those around you? Maybe those incentives drive you to some extent, but personally I believe that success is much more about the joy you get from your job. The happiness you receive when you're in the swing of work or the satisfaction you get from seeing your hard work gain momentum. I have met and know quite a few people who are considered 'successful'. They have reached the headiest of heights in their chosen fields, have gained respect from their peers, have possibly earned great sums of money, are known as 'powerful' and at times lead the way, but do THEY feel successful? Some of them do because they love their job but some most definitely do not. I have been witness to people like this, who to the outside world are the stereotype of 'success' career-wise, but who actually feel empty as they assumed there would be some sort of enlightened freedom at the end of working their way to the top. Reaching the 'top' doesn't mean you are immune to pain, stress and discomfort in life. It doesn't excuse you from the stresses that loss, bereavement or illness leave behind. Money can of course alleviate a certain amount of stress – when bills are mounting up and there are family members to feed, that anxiety is all-consuming. Having financial security may at times ease this pressure and slow the ever-spinning hamster wheel of work, but having buckets of money, power or a tonne of accolades doesn't mean you'll be able to protect yourself from the tensions that life throws your way. You cannot buy deep-rooted clarity or calm.

I grew up with two parents who worked extremely hard to make sure my brother, Jamie, and I were fed, clothed and had the odd fun trip away. My dad worked most days as a sign writer and still does to this day, whilst my mum continuously cared for us on top of juggling several jobs as an orthodontist nurse, clothes delivery driver and part-time cleaner for our neighbours. I had no grasp, as a kid, of the sacrifices my parents made to ensure we had a level of security and comfort, but boy do I now! Their tenacity has also instilled in me a work ethic that I cannot ignore. I have seen first-hand how hard work can bring you so much joy and with it calm. My dad still works up to six days a week as a sign writer, even though he has no children to worry about any more he continues to put in the hours because he adores his job. That right there is success. His career has spanned close to five decades and has allowed him a great creative flow and sense of purpose that he still holds on to today.

I guess what I'm trying to say is, you can own the flash cars, you can wear the tailored suits, you can hobnob with the it-gang but it doesn't guarantee that nourishing feeling of success – and continually looking for it or feeling like we should be doing better than we are can be a great cause of stress. Finding your own groove, engaging with the job at hand or people you work with on a deeper level will make for a satisfied and calm mind when you go to bed at night. You don't have to have a high-powered career or fancy job to reap the rewards of this comfort. You just have to get the best out of the job you do.

Whatever your job, make your own markers of success; be honest and authentic in what you do – this will help you down the path to calm.

PRESSURE TO DO BETTER

If you feel a heavy weight bearing down on you, to be better or do better at work, can you route back to where that pressure comes from? I certainly can within my own working life. I might try to convince myself it comes from wanting to please my parents, or to prove to certain naysayers that I'm better than they imagined, or even that I'm trying to show my children how a good work ethic is achieved but I know deep down, below all the surface fog of thoughts and chat, that it is ME. I'm the only one who is applying such a force and pressure to be better, move faster, be smarter and apply myself more. I'm not even sure why these pressures are there but it feels relatively unstoppable and engine-powered. I'm my worst critic. I'm the most judgmental when it comes to my cock-ups and I'm the one who needs to see tangible proof to believe I am good enough.

These thoughts and pressures can push me far from calm, but as long as I take a minute to remember they're all coming from ME I can take the heat off the situation somewhat and start to give myself a break. It doesn't matter if I wasn't stumble-free and perfect on the radio. The world won't shatter if I didn't pronounce a word correctly on a broadcast and no one cares if I wasn't cited as the best that day. It's all an illusion anyway. A view of opinions somehow stitched together to form some sort of answer to a nonsensical equation.

Remember to give yourself a break! Don't beat yourself up when the pressure is on. If something goes wrong, take a deep breath, learn from it and let it pass. Easier said than done, but there's not much point stressing about something that has been and gone and that you can't do anything about now. All you'll be doing is growing yourself a little bud of stress. If we turn over our mistakes again and again in our minds they seem bigger, but if we do the opposite they can fade naturally with time. Be kind to yourself – route back to what I talked about earlier in the book; think about what you'd say to a friend. What you'd more than likely say is 'It doesn't matter – forget about it.'

TAKE FIVE

Try to make time and space for thoughts and ideas – even if you're ridiculously busy – as that is where the calm will find you. It doesn't need to be a huge stretch of time, and you can fit it around other things you'll definitely do in the day. When you go to the loo, when you make tea, when you go to grab lunch, when you are sitting down and eating – at any of these points, use five minutes to not do anything. Close your eyes and perhaps do some of the breathing exercises from page 63. Use the time to clear your mind so that you can make space for thoughts, ideas and calm to climb in. By giving yourself a mental breather from your immediate work stresses, you'll gain perspective and clarity to then tackle those hurdles in a calmer way.

Just as there is no room for calm when work is non-stop, equally there is no home for it if energies stay stagnant and immovable for too long. If you feel that you're not fulfilling your full potential and you've lost the rhythm to make leaps and changes, try another way. I've hit dead ends in my career so many times. I've been told I'm not 'quite right' for jobs (whatever that means), felt misunderstood and also personally felt like I wasn't doing my best. These are always moments where I've taken a step back to look at everything going on around me. Why am I not doing my best and why do I care if others think I'm not good enough? This might lead to change or thinking about things differently.

At times I've felt an urge to learn a little more. I always feel calm when I'm letting new information swamp my brain. Is there room in your job, or outside of work, to learn more? I think there probably always is in most jobs or hobbies.

At other times I'll look to see if I can be a help or positive force for someone else. Helping another is always so fulfilling and calming because you reach your

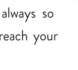

full potential immediately. At times I've pined for change and a new challenge. When I get bored or complacent, although I'm using up less energy, I do not feel calm at all, I feel fidgety and irritated. Challenging yourself is always fun if you're doing it for the right reasons. Don't heap challenges on yourself to be the best out there, beat others or get praise; do it because you know deep down it'll awaken your soul and make you feel zingy and in the moment again. When I'm faced with a challenge I feel very alive and very in the moment, which usually always leads me back to calm. No one out there can stop you looking for new challenges. Remember, they don't have to be huge, just something that's new to you! The great thing is you create them and decide when it's time to give them a go.

I often swing between two extremes – of feeling overwhelmed and a bit stuck – and I know calm cannot live in either of these spaces. I am always on the lookout for great expansive gaps where calm can set up shop or necessary movement to help calmly energise my dreams and ideas. Don't be scared of silence and space. I find this one hard, too, but I'm learning to love the distant hum of detachment from everything that I usually allow to consume me. Find those moments and snatches of time and space where you can recalibrate and recharge.

Summary

FIND YOUR BALANCE.

THINK OUTSIDE THE BOX.

DEFINE YOUR OWN SUCCESS.

Whether you love or hate work, make sure there's time for you too.

Don't be afraid to change things up if you need to.

Don't worry about everyone else, aim for what will keep YOU fulfilled.

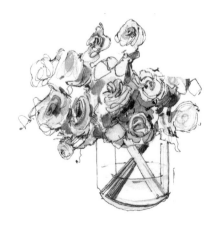

WHAT DOES CALM WORK LOOK LIKE TO YOU?

Write one word or draw a picture here that sums it up.

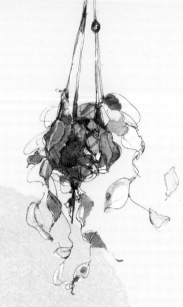

CALM ENVIRONMENT

Can you think of a place that makes you instantly deeply exhale? A place that can draw out all stresses and tensions as soon as you step foot in its space? A place where you feel grounded, safe and, most importantly, calm? I have a few of these heavenly spots that spring to mind and when I even think of them a small wave of serenity washes over me. The first is a clearing in the woods near to my house. Giant trees dwarf me and remind me of scale and perspective. Their history and stability brings me a rooted calm that makes me stop in my tracks.

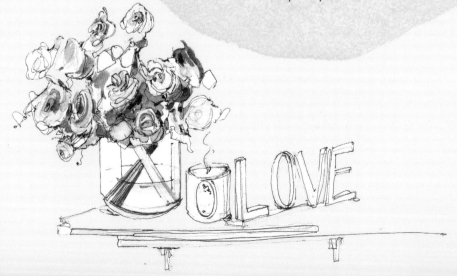

MAGIC PLACES

When I was pregnant with Honey I was consumed with a combination of what felt like food poisoning and sea sickness. Some days the sickness was so intense I felt helpless and trapped. I would waddle over to this shady spot and lie in the branches of one of the huge fallen trees, letting its knots and gnarls cradle me and my queasiness. I could see the blue sky through the tree tops and for a moment everything would stop spinning. It's now a spot where I love to take the children to so we can all bask in the energy of those giant oaks.

Another place I can slip into this chilled-out state is one of my old friend's houses. There is something weirdly magical about the location and energy trapped between its walls that sucks me in and makes me feel at home. I spent a lot of my carefree teenage years in this house, so muscle memory encourages me into a freer-spirited and fun version of myself and my worries seem to slip away.

Another calm place for me is by the sea. I'm sure most of you will agree that there is something hypnotic and wild yet impossibly calming about being in its view. Not only is the ocean visually bewildering and beautiful in any of its varying states, but energetically there is an inexplicable force behind its draw. Suddenly any overriding emotions are blown apart and shattered by the crashing waves and magnetic pull. Even when it's pissing down, it's still bewitching to be near. I can't think of many other places that have the ability to still look and feel great on a cloudy Tuesday.

On one short trip away with my husband before we had Rex and Honey, the weather was slightly overcast and the sea quite choppy. There was a small plateau in a

Calm spaces don't have to be a long haul flight away or anywhere fancy at all. It's all about creating an atmosphere that feels right to you.

Is there a space in your house that feels calm? ....

What colours make you feel calm? ....

Does that space need a clear-out to create more space? ....

Brainstorm some ideas of how you can make that space your own utopia:

....

....

....

....

....

....

....

nearby rock formation that led perfectly into a deeper part of the ocean. The thought of getting into those churning waves was, at first, beyond unappealing, but after a few friends braved the chill, we decided to follow suit. The initial shock of the unfavourable temperature was soon vanquished by a feeling of liberation. Every nerve ending in my body woke up and made every colour, smell and sensation heighten within seconds. I could hear the wind whipping about my hair and feel the salt sticking to my face as unruly waves chopped about my cheeks. Being thrown about and bobbing ferociously up and down was exciting and uncertain yet felt weirdly comforting and safe at the same time. Every bit of my body and soul loved being in that water and the feeling lasted some time afterwards. Unfortunately I don't live by the sea so I don't get this experience enough, but I guess that also makes those moments that bit sweeter when they do happen.

None of these places or spaces are exclusive, fancy or particularly out of the ordinary. What they are, though, is magic. They hold a powerful force that draws me in and makes me feel rooted, at home and very calm.

So what is it about these places that has the ability to quash any feelings of stress or discomfort for me? I believe it's a full-bodied concoction of many sensations and energies in that place that make my own energy feel aligned and supported. Energy is such a tough one to put our fingers on because it is not tangible or visible in any way. It's a feeling, a vibe, an atmosphere. More often than not, I think it's just a magic that comes from the natural state of the area. For example, the sea and all of its negative ions. Negative ions have the power to increase our mood, improve our senses and can even provide relief from pain. The energy of the falling waves causes the splitting of neutral particles of air, freeing electrons which then latch onto other air molecules, causing a negative charge. This is why we get an instant boost from being by the sea. All of those negative ions allow our senses to awaken, our bodies to physically benefit all round and our minds to calm.

There are many magical locations on planet Earth that have a magnetic pull, such as Stonehenge, in Britain, or Es Vedrà, in Ibiza. These parts of the Earth are steeped in a magnetic energy that can have positive health-altering and healing powers. After all, the magnetic field which spreads outwards from Earth's interior protects our planet and our ozone layer and has a lot more bearing on all of us than we care to give time to. Therefore these magic spots on Earth which exhibit such magnetism act as a reminder of how powerful the natural energies on our planet are. We tend to assume all comfort and calming must come from something attained or reached, but more often than not it lies in the hands of nature and simplicity.

If you feel wired, fatigued by stress or simply a little all over the shop, head outside. Is there a park or a green spot near you or a nice tree to sit under? Find your own peaceful spot and make it yours. No one has to know, no signpost or painted spot needs to mark your territory, just know it's yours inside.

Nature can instantly remind us of calm, as it carries on evolving, growing and changing when everything else feels completely chaotic. Trees keep on growing when we feel out of control, birds keep on singing when we are lost in stress, and the sea keeps on rolling when we feel rock bottom. This is a great gentle reminder that the world will keep turning even when we feel torn apart by stress and pressure. Get outside and soak it all up. The sounds, the smells, the feel of the breeze on your skin. For me, this is instant calm.

NOSTALGIC PLACES

As well as these natural wonders we can use to access calm, are the joyful places to which we have attached memory and nostalgia. These are locations where good times have been had and happy thoughts live on. I'm naturally very nostalgic so this idea is a powerful one for me. Visiting a place where something traumatic or upsetting has happened affects me greatly and I find it very tricky to get my calm back. I'm hugely sensitive to the energy of spaces like this and find it hard to shake off these feelings for some time. But the reverse is equally as impactful; places that I have packed out with gorgeous, hazy memories remain some of my favourite spots for feeling calm. I think it can be relatively damaging to live vividly in the past, as we then forget to act from the NOW, but when it comes to routing back to your own place of calm, recalling happy memories in happy spaces can have hugely positive effects.

If you have ever moved from one property to another you may have noticed how after a short while your new space feels like home. Once the upheaval and chaos of a move begins to dissipate and once loved ones have left their own imprint in your new dwelling, it starts to feel more YOU. I believe that each happy memory that occurs in that new space and each person who enters the door leaves a bit of energy that then lives on and becomes part of your home. The new space becomes softer, warmer and more comforting and pockets will remain within those walls that bring you calm. For me, it's one end of my kitchen where a small sofa lines up to a window that overlooks a church. Over the last few years we have crammed our kitchen with people we adore; laughing, eating and leaving their own mark. The energy that flows around that space feels fun and frenetic but supportive and calm, too. When the kids are in bed and I've loaded the dishwasher I like to lie on that sofa and read books with one eye on the view out of the window. The night sky frames the scene and I feel calm knowing that I am safe and comforted.

All our other senses come into play when we seek out these peaceful places. Are there smells or colours that you know instantly relax each muscle in your body? Back in my twenties my dear friend Lolly and I went on a girls' holiday to Mexico. We were both experiencing very chaotic portions of our lives, with me fresh out of a broken engagement and Lolly holding down a frantic job managing a busy nightclub in London. On the ride to the airport I remember Lolly wondering how she would have a whole seven days away from her two ever-chirping phones. What if she let everyone down? What if the whole business crumbled in that time? What if, what if... It was exhausting to even contemplate as we were both approaching a subconsciously pivotal point in our lives.

The first seminal moment of this trip revolved solely around smell. We were welcomed by some very smiley faces who took our over-packed suitcases from us and began wafting incense around our frazzled bodies. What was this intoxicating smell and how on earth was it filtering into every stressed nook in my system? From that point onwards we had seven days of total, relaxed and calm bliss. I asked the front desk for some of that heavenly incense for our room and then continued to burn it day and night. I wondered if this smell would only take hold in a paradise setting but it seemed to have the same effect back on British shores. When I got down to the last stick of incense I felt completely bereft. How could I not have this go-to calming smell in my life anymore? I had no idea where to buy it as it was local produce from the Mexican coastline we stayed on. Two years later I was in a market in Ibiza with my kids when this rush of nostalgia hit me straight in the solar plexus. A full-bodied sensation of calm and joy. It was THE smell. I rushed back along this trail of scent, desperately seeking out a stall that could facilitate my calming habit, then BOOM... I spotted two older Mexican men adorned with silver rings and patchwork boots who had a beautifully decorated stall of local crafts and THE incense. JACKPOT! I bought every last packet and practically skipped home beaming with joy. Lolly and I have since used up every single stick of the stuff, so I'm sitting patiently until I get to that wonderful little market in Ibiza one of these days.

Who would have thought smell could be such a game changer? Maybe it's not for everyone but for me it instantly evokes memories and feelings that have an impactful power over my body and mind. Certain perfumes from my childhood make me feel safe and supported as they remind me of my mum. The smell of strong paint makes me feel more grounded and connected as it takes me back to watching my dad sign-write in his workshop when I was small. For me, this simple intoxicating sensory trip will always route me back to calm, if only for a short while. Try to find your favourite, meaningful scent, it could just the trick that sets you on your way for a calmer day.

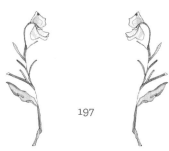

BRINGING CALM HOME

Colour is equally as powerful for me in the calm stakes. Our bedroom at home is mostly white. For me, white equals tranquility. It helps my mind stop whirring and makes my body feel relaxed. Our bedroom needs to have this soothing quality as I don't always sleep well, so whatever it takes to help me relax after a busy day is a must. Other parts of my house are injected with colour as there is less need for serenity in those places. Our front room is a concoction of dusty pink and moss green, which makes it feel soothing yet still fun, as that is a place where we gather as a family and play, chat and watch TV. Our kitchen has pops of pink and turquoise because it is the engine room of the house. It's where we are constantly cooking, chatting and organising our family life. Our bathroom is also white as it spells winding down for the day for us and the kids. It's the first pit-stop on route to the land of 'Z's, so it needs to embody that placidity that can carry us on to a good night's sleep.

Getting our surroundings to reflect the calm we want to be feeling inside can be a powerful tool, but it doesn't need to mean a huge DIY redecoration project. My husband is very good at mood lighting, which might make him sound like some kind of 70s smoothie, but really we both find it incredibly important for the evening wind-down. His mother was all about the magic of lighting, so she instilled in him this need for mood-changing lamps and candles. Nothing out of the ordinary or fancy, just some good old-fashioned candlelight and a twist of the dimmer switch. This sort of atmosphere switch up can really help set the tone for an evening, whether you have people over or are in for a night of blissful solitude. Our brains most definitely pick up on this sort of obvious signpost and act accordingly. Our brains know, perhaps by some sort of prehistoric recall, that less light equals winding down. There is a lot that has been written about how our phone screens, laptops and computers emanate a blue light which strips us of melatonin, the hormone that is needed for sleep, and I know that if I stay up too late writing on my laptop the light which emanates from the screen makes for a night of hellish interrupted sleep. Just last week whilst writing this book I pushed on into the later hours and then was completely wired until 2a.m. As somebody who a) loves sleep and b) has kids who are fond of waking around 6am, this was bad news. I started to almost panic that I would never sleep again. Sleep deprivation is not only annoying when it's happening but also stops you from thinking rationally. Ever heard of the term 'baby brain'? It isn't so much a flimsy concept where us shattered mums blame our kids for lack of sleep, it really refers to the fact that we cannot string a sentence together as our minds are much more jumbled without the desired eight hours of sleep.

The right lighting can help us feel calm after a busy day, set the scene for romance, energise us if exhausted and top up our happiness on a sunny day. It's instant, easily achieved and really does work. I think that making yourself a calm space for some solitary serenity or a group gathering is really important as you want the energy to be right for a peaceful yet lovely time. It's of course not just about lighting, there are many little things you can do that can set the scene for your mind to get the cue to relax and wind down.

DECLUTTERING OUR ENVIRONMENTS

As I'm sure you are all by now well aware, I'm a complete neat freak. I have a tedious habit of continuously scanning my house for things that are out of place. I have probably taken this one to the extreme, but to me, tidy house, tidy head. There is no way I could sit down after the kids are in bed to start writing if there was a sink full of dishes and Lego all over the floor. My mind would feel jumbled, chaotic and not ready to calmly write. I think most of the time the general state of our homes relates back to our personalities, or how we feel deep down. My need for cleanliness and control 100 per cent reflects how I often feel very out of control. I feel that life's chaotic tendencies spin me out so much that I have to cling onto the small amounts of control that I do have. Keeping my house in order makes me subconsciously believe I have more of a hold on life's plan than I actually do. I can at least trick my brain in to a calmer state by creating a calm and controlled environment at home.

I do believe that we can lean into that chaos at times and feel calm in it, as I mentioned back in the Family chapter, but my theory is that the energy in the house can't flow as it is meant to with objects and mess scattered around. I'm no feng shui master but I recognise when my house feels at bursting point and when I need a good old tidy up and a clear-out. I try to have a bit of a declutter every few months, because with my kids' and step-kids' ever-increasing hoard, plus mine and my husband's love of clothes, we need to let stuff go to allow the new in. I'm not talking about loads of new acquisitions necessarily, just newness in the form of energy and opportunity. I think that if we are emotionally holding on to loads of objects in our homes we are stopping the necessary flow of life, and it is often a sign that we are a little stuck in the past. Of course we will all have possessions in our lives that represent a lot of meaning and will never be parted with, I'm talking more about holding on to things we know we don't really need or that are actually causing us more pain than joy. I'm constantly trying to declutter but in the velocity of modern life I don't always have the time I need to thoroughly look at our home and what we actually need.

But when you go on holiday, you realise how little you really need to get by. A few outfits, some toiletries and you're good to go. At home we seem to believe we need so much more than we actually do. I know that after I've had a good run through the house with a bin bag for the charity shop, I feel like I have much more clarity and headspace.

The other wonderful thing about having a clear-out is that you will more than likely benefit others in the process. My mum puts on a little yard sale at hers a few times a year where she has collected bits and bobs from family and friends that are no longer needed. She has a fun gathering with cake and tea and her friends and neighbours buy up things they like the look of for a bargain price. All of that money then goes to an animal charity as she is hugely passionate about helping those causes. As well as adding to my mum's charity sale loot, I give a lot to my local charity shop, knowing that the things in my home that no longer serve a purpose will bring happiness to someone else as well as aid the chosen charity. WIN WIN! Less clutter in your home, less clutter in your mind as well as helping other people out there.

HELLO TO . . . ALICE AND LAURA

Creating a calm space is of paramount importance for two friends of mine who regularly host supper clubs for groups of excited strangers. Alice Levine and Laura Jackson are not only brilliant broadcasters on our screens and on radios but they're also the hostesses with the mostesses . . . Wait, that doesn't work, but you get my point. They've been friends for years and both love cooking and entertaining, so they started up their own supper club which they do for fun alongside their careers. Their inventive food concoctions teamed with their delicate eye for all-round comfort and class has won over tonnes of feasted fans. Their supper clubs are visually fairytale gorgeous with Pinterest-board-worthy table settings, soft candlelight and colour palettes that instantly relax. Who better to hit up for some advice on how to set the scene for a relaxed and calm evening?

"

F: Hello ladies, how are you? I'm constantly in awe of your supper clubs and how beautiful they are. Every inch of your gatherings look elegant, chic and so very calming. How did you start out creating these nights?

A: It all began as a challenge – can we open a 'restaurant' for the night in Laura's flat and have 20 people come and eat? Can we make it look great and taste great? Can we make people feel like they've had a completely unique experience?

L: We normally start with the season as a 'theme', that way we can ensure that we are using the freshest ingredients for the food, as seasonality and provenance is really important to us. With the season defining the food, we also look into what flowers are in around that time too, using their colours as a base for the evening in terms of tablecloths and tableware.

F: What is the main aim when you are organising one of your nights?

A: People having a good time is definitely the main aim. The food, of course, is important and the space and the table looking eye-catching and inviting is key, but mainly we want people to go home at the end of the evening saying they've had fun and met some great people.

L: We love to bring different people together, as food really unites people of all different walks of life. You can get the most diverse, interesting people around a kitchen table with a plate of food and it unites everyone around it. It's really powerful. We aim to bring people together through their shared love of food, to chat and enjoy a night of laughter with new friends.

F: As well as delicious food, how important is the setting and colour palette for your evenings?

A: We play around with colour a lot. We've done serene schemes using mainly white (the napkins, tablecloth, crockery etc.) with the addition of a subtle pop of colour from dusty pink hydrangeas, for example. Or we've gone for something moodier with indigo linen and raffia place mats.

L: We spend a lot of time looking for fabrics, place mats and vintage crockery so that each evening we devise feels special. It makes the guests feel so valued when they each have their own personalised place setting – all the little extras go a really long way.

F: Which colours do you find calming when you're working out the scheme for an evening?

A: Pale, plain and neutral don't have to be the only ways to do calming – we've had dusty pink blush tones, dove grey and navy as the main palette, but we love to go bolder and brighter with clashing prints, too, which can be equally inviting.

L: I think nothing too busy, something really clean, simple and chic is always very calming. Light pastel colours I would say have the most calming effect, and if you're feeling like adding a pop of colour it's easy to do so with candlesticks, platters or even gold cutlery.

F: As well as colour, what else is important for getting the right mood?

A: Lighting. No one has ever had a lovely time sat under a 100-watt bulb in the central light. Use incidental lighting with lamps and candles.
And music – silence can make people feel edgy but blaring tunes can stop people from chatting freely, so volume is as important as the music choice itself.

L: Music and lighting are key for creating the perfect mood. Lighting needs to be candlelight or low-level lamps, no bright overhead light bulbs and no spotlights. Music needs to be loud enough so that it creates a little buzz, but quiet enough for people to talk over. My favourite two fail-safe, easy listening soundtracks are from the films *Dirty Dancing* and *Amelie.*

F: How do you both keep calm in the chaos of having to cook and cater for big numbers?

L: Well, there are times when we do not feel calm at all, but it's so lovely working together because we help each other to feel relaxed even when it can be really stressful. Before guests come we normally take 10 minutes to do our make-up and get dressed out of our cooking clothes. These few minutes allow us to 'get in the zone'.

F: Thank you so much ladies! When can I come for tea?

SPRING-CLEANING THE PAST

There are some objects in my house that don't bring me that much joy and I know I'm holding on to for the wrong reasons. Perhaps you are holding on to gifts that an ex-partner gave you because mentally you haven't fully let go of the relationship? Maybe you're clinging on to certain possessions because you didn't have much growing up? Maybe you cannot let go of your belongings because you feel they make up such a big part of who you are?

I did something very therapeutic yet possibly quite reckless a few years ago when I felt I needed to move on from stagnant energy and open up to newness. I had written a diary most weeks since a very young age, and there were 50 or so notepads sat under my bed like a treasure chest of memories, adventures, traumas and tears. As well as holding many secrets and wonderful stories, these books made me feel heavy. They felt too rigid and one-dimensional. They were stories told at one particular time when I felt very differently to how I do today. I felt burdened by these books and their words, so I spontaneously set about burning them all. Thousands of words went up in flames, losing their weight and hold on my life. Maybe it would have been massively fun to look over them all when I'm old and wizened, but maybe they were holding me back, too. Maybe they were making me believe my story defined who I am now and these stories had actually had reached their expiry date. It felt worth the gamble and I don't regret it one bit at this point in time. The house feels lighter and clearer without them in my life and I still have loads of memories in my head to flick back to if and when I choose. Letting go is tough but sometimes it can be game-changing and beyond liberating. I think subconsciously I was also ready for new stories to be told that weren't hindered by my visions of the past. New patterns of thinking and a calmer outlook on the future.

THE POWER OF PEN AND PAPER

I also have the tendency to feel overwhelmed with running our home. Keeping the cogs turning within family life and making sure everyone is happy and has what they need can often take up so much time and energy when there feels like there is none. Our house is always full of energy, people and things that seemingly need fixing. There is always a floppy shelf, broken loo seat or loose tap in our house. As I said, I like things organised so the list of things that need replacing, fixing or restoring is endless. The only method I have found that works in these out-of-control moments is to write lists. It's the most basic and dull of hobbies but one that makes me feel in check. I have several notepads that are always in my handbag and often contain lines like:

- Water plants
- Fix loo seat (again)
- Replace dead plants
- Buy loo roll
- Sort out kids' clothes.

Once pen has hit paper and that idea or thought has been made permanent I can let it leave my brain forever. More space, more clarity and more calm.

I used to think it terribly tragic that my mum was forever writing lists when I was

We all hoard and hold on to certain objects, photos, or items of clothing because we have emotional attachment to them. Some people find letting go of stuff very traumatic and it can hold them back hugely. Others simply need to really think about what they need and want in their personal space and perhaps just a little time to actually sort through it all.

Write in the sack below what you know you're holding on to – is there anything in there that you don't need that you could give away?

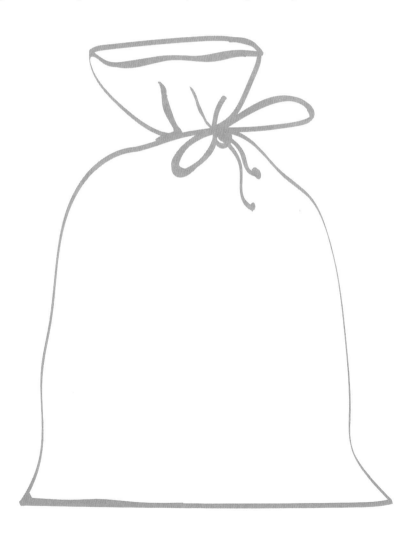

a kid but I have most definitely taken up this pasttime and run with it. I would be lost without them. I'm much more likely to keep on top of things at home whilst managing to keep my cool if I have my nerdy notebook nearby. If your head feels full, why not give this trick a go too?

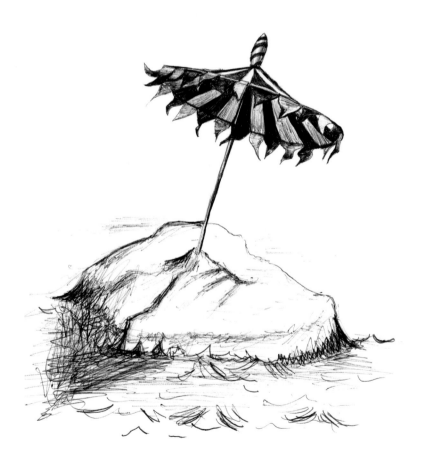

Music is always my biggest remedy and healer when I'm feeling stressed. I let songs drench me and revive me and I love their healing power. These songs always bring me back to my place of calm! Here is my calm playlist. What is yours? Write your list below.

MY CALM PLAYLIST

Sampha – 'Too Much'

George Harrison – 'My Sweet Lord'

Baz Luhrmann – 'Everybody's Free (To Wear Sunscreen)'

Neil Young – 'Razor Love'

Bon Iver – '29 #Strafford APTS'

Elton John – 'Mellow'

Fleet Foxes – 'Blue Ridge Mountains'

Oasis – 'Champagne Supernova'

Tracy Chapman – 'For You'

Groove Armada – 'At the river'

Laura Mvula – 'She'

Led Zeppelin – 'The Rain Song'

Otis Redding – '(Sittin' On) The Dock of the Bay'

Bat For Lashes – 'Travelling Woman'

Bob Marley – 'Three Little Birds'

Chris Stapleton – 'Traveller'

Nick Mulvey – 'Mountain to Move'

London Grammar – 'Rooting For You'

YOUR CALM PLAYLIST

HELLO TO . . . KATE

For advice on how to declutter, I thought I'd speak to expert Kate Ibbotson.

F: Kate, you're a professional declutterer, what exactly does this entail?

K: I work one-to-one with clients who are struggling with clutter and disorganisation – in their homes and workspaces on the surface but in their lives and minds when we delve deeper. The process is quite structured:

- I start by helping them create a vision for their space by honing in on their unique style and personality type.
- Then the physical declutter takes place through questioning whether an item adds true value to their life compared to the space it takes up.
- I put in place organisational systems, routines and appropriate storage which ensures the smooth running of their house.
- I have links with different charities, i.e. homeless shelters, food banks and animal charities so I can donate almost any item on the client's behalf.

We don't just address the physical stuff – everyone carries around mental and emotional clutter, so a big part of my job is coaxing out the reasons why clients accumulate things or fail to let things go.

F: How much do you think the space around us impacts our state of mind?

K: There's no doubt that living in a mess can lead to stress. Being surrounded by lots of physical possessions can bombard the senses and drain energy. I also don't believe it's possible to relax at the end of the day in a cluttered home. This environment would send signals to the brain that there is still work to do, and it creates anxiety because it feels like such a huge mountain to climb.

Clutter has other negative effects which can increase general stress levels. Time – surely the most precious commodity we have – can be lost searching for misplaced possessions, and it also costs money. It's very common to buy a duplicate of something if a possession is misplaced. I also regularly see people buy more possessions to make themselves feel better about living in a cluttered home.

Possibly the most insidious cost of clutter, though, is the guilt and embarrassment it can bring upon people. This may cause a reluctance to invite others into the home, or anxiety when visitors are due or when people drop by unannounced.

In contrast, when we surround ourselves with possessions we find useful and/or beautiful and when we follow simple systems for maintaining order, we not only feel inspired and energised, we also give ourselves more opportunity for psychological growth. For example, we might feel creative and start a project and we are more productive because of lower stress levels and fewer distractions. People even report that relationships improve, they make healthier food and lifestyle choices and they sleep better – all because of exerting positive control over their environment.

F: What are the reasons why people find it hard to create order and clear stuff at home?

K: The number one reason for failing to create order is having too much stuff in the first place. We need to streamline and simplify first because otherwise we could be organising forever. But we also need to think, 'Why do we have too much stuff?'

Older members of society often have the 'make do and mend' post-war mentality ingrained in them which younger people inherit. Taking care of belongings saves money and encourages an appreciation of them, but the concept can be taken too far. Some people hang on to duplicates or possessions which don't work properly or are no longer to their taste.

There's also the rise of cheap retail. There's nothing inherently wrong with cheap goods (if they were made ethically) but people tend to end up with a larger volume of goods because of the low price tag. And the rise of cheap retail MIXED with a waste-not want-not mentality is a very cluttered combination.

Sellers want us to be happy with our purchase, but very soon afterwards they want us to be dissatisfied! They wouldn't make any money if we were content in the long term. Most people aren't immune to clever marketing and at some point they have been sucked in by hype.

A psychological theory could shed some light on why one purchase tends to lead to another. The Diderot effect refers to the process whereby a purchase or gift creates dissatisfaction with existing possessions and environment, provoking a potentially spiralling pattern of consumption. An example would be buying a new sofa and then wanting a new coffee table to match.

Another simple explanation for rising levels of possessions might be that these days the population takes for granted entire classes of possessions that didn't exist in years gone by. Children's toys tend to be marketed with an end game to 'collect them all'. Electronics come with various add-ons and wires/cables (isn't it so common to have drawers full of these things?). More products have simply been invented. All this contributes to cluttered homes.

People also gather stuff to soothe and protect themselves, relying on it for confidence, authority, escapism, freedom and fun. Possessions are clearly something everyone needs but there is a limit. If we don't feel 'good enough' internally, 'things' are just a cover-up for our insecurities. The truth is, we can't buy contentment, we have to cultivate it ourselves – from within – otherwise it's just trying to fill a hole that can never be filled.

F: What are your own rules about clearing out?

K: I follow some pretty simple rules. I find that, once the initial full-house declutter is done, they are quick and easy to follow:

- Being intentional about what I buy. I love shopping but if I have even the tiniest doubt about a purchase, I won't make it, because I know it's going to end up as clutter. If unsure, I'll exercise a 'purchase pause' – holding off and seeing how I feel in a week.
- Assign a home to each possession. Everything within the house will have a permanent resting place. It helps to use drawer dividers and storage containers for smaller items, and labelling can work well, too.
- I keep a large bag in the understairs cupboard specifically for charity shop donations. When I realise something is surplus to requirements, it goes straight in there. With a

family of four, I find that around a bin liner per month goes out – I think of my home as having a turnover!

- Each possession has to add value to life in some way. Either because it's useful – like a potato peeler – or because it makes me smile – like a handwritten note or piece of art. If an item holds a negative memory or I can find something else to do the same job, I'd rather have the space it takes up instead.
- Return possessions to their 'home' after use. This will reduce the need for constant tidying up. I follow the mantra: 'don't put it down, put it away'.
- I don't buy in bulk. I try to use up toiletries and food in the freezer. I figure that the worst that can happen is that I have to pop out to a shop for something essential and it's easier to keep track of what I have this way.

F: How do you work with someone who is emotionally hoarding objects/clothing/paperwork?

K: It's not as simple as just getting them to have a clear-out. I get to the root of why they can't let go or why they are accumulating too much. Are they a perfectionist? Does this stem from not feeling good enough? Are they delaying making a decision about an item? Does this stem from anxiety? Do they feel unfulfilled so they are looking to possessions to provide that excitement? I always start by dealing with less-emotional possessions such as the contents of a kitchen drawer. We then work our way up to books, clothes and sentimental items.

F: What should we be aiming for to create a calm environment at home?

K: It's important to have a clear vision in mind. So I recommend looking for inspiration in magazines or online. What the individual's personality is like or what their hobbies are will determine what storage is most appropriate. It's important that the furniture chosen is not too big for the rooms as this can cause a cluttered feel. Wall storage, furniture that doubles up for another use and adding shelving can all make a massive difference. Possessions should be easy to reach and stored near to where we use them – this will mean we're more likely to return them to their place after use.

UNCALM PLACES

 So we know that calm spaces exist for us and we know that we are capable of creating our own magic spots, but what about when you have to enter places that feel overwhelming? How do we find the calm within that chaos? I struggle with this one a lot and constantly strive to get better at carving my own patch of stillness within the madness. My husband and I are both slightly uncomfortable at big, loud parties. Jesse doesn't drink so he can't even opt to get inebriated to relax into the throes of a crowd. My overbearing feelings are of paranoia. I panic at what I'm saying and how I'm coming across and feel instantly uncool and transparent. I assume everyone else feels self-assured and confident whereas I may be putting on a smile and chatting to new faces, but I feel everyone else can see every mistake I've ever made. It feels as though they all have x-ray vision and can see past the smile and make-up to the holes in my own story. There will be times when I go out and for no particular reason feel more confident than normal and so slot into a crowd with much more ease and comfort. I love it when this happens, but more often than not I just feel awkward. Busy environments tend to take me out of my calm space and make me feel like I'm having a slight out-of-body experience, as I try to keep up with conversation while avoiding any trip-ups or awkward moments like potholes in the road.

 In these moments I try to take a step back, and rather than let my motormouth spiral out of control in panic, I just breathe and let these moments occur naturally, and as they need to. In conversation I'll try to ask questions rather than talk at someone, which also helps to remove the heat and attention from the imagined impending doom. If someone looks like they aren't that interested in talking to me I'll work out a way to politely leave the situation to find my calm somewhere else.

Of course, there are times when slipping into the chaos can be quite fun. As long as you plan to get back to your calm place later on, dipping your toe into waters you know are too deep for you can be rather exhilarating. If I'm at a work event where I feel out of my depth, because I'm surrounded by well-known faces or people who are seemingly powerful, rather than extracting myself from the energy of it altogether I'll sometimes dare myself to get a little closer. Or perhaps I'm at a wedding where I only know two other people. Rather than hug them closely whilst necking Pimm's, I'll dare myself to go and talk to people I've never met before. It may feel wildly unnatural and slightly unnerving but in this territory there is a lot to learn about ourselves. It's getting that balance between feeling content enough to be open to learn yet courageous enough to step out of our own comfort zones.

With my weird job I have leapt out of my comfort zone on so many occasions and have felt millions of miles away from my calm spot. I have interviewed people who have such charisma and confidence that I have felt minuscule and I have broadcast from places where chaos felt rife and uncontrollable. In these circumstances I have leaned into the chaos and learned a lot about myself whilst having a lot of fun along the way. These moments are also an opportunity to remember that we are all the same. When we end up in a group of people we feel very different to it can feel chaotic. We may feel alienated or uncomfortable, but by talking to new faces we realise quickly that we are all the same deep down. We all have the capabilities to love, grow and change and that knowledge is deeply calming. Losing the feeling of being different or out of place allows us to relax in new places and situations with a little more ease.

Getting back to the calm after experiencing a bit of fun and chaos isn't always easy but I usually get there in the end via a combination of time and thought. I usually have a bad night's sleep after a new high-energy job as I try desperately to process all the new feelings and emotions and words spoken, so that I can start to crawl back to calm. There is definitely a window of time where I am quite literally shaking off the energies of new people and new places that I've experienced that day. My head will rattle through the day's highs and lows and try to make sense of it all so I can begin to let go of it and go to sleep. The next day I will still have the afterglow of having stepped out of my comfort zone but I'll also be that bit closer to calm.

If being in busy spaces makes you nervous, or having new people around derails you somewhat, always try to route back to the knowledge that it doesn't matter what others think of you. If I'm out with my children and one of them has a tantrum it can feel completely catastrophic and embarrassing at the time. I will more than likely be red-faced, moving at high speed and desperately trying to shrink to minimise any personal damage. I don't want to look like a failure or be judged by others, so I lose my calm altogether. If in those moments I can step back and find my own peaceful spot within my own environment, breathe and remember it doesn't matter what other people's judgments are, I'll be okay. In these moments where we feel wildly out of control we must try to go within and just deal with what is going on for us while blocking out the scene around us. We cannot get back to a grounded place if our

If you feel stressed out in busy places, repeat a simple sentence in your head that allows you to focus on getting back to your place of calm. What is your personal calming mantra?

MY MANTRA

I am safe, I am loved

YOUR MANTRA

eyes and minds are wandering too far from our own hearts. I think in this day and age we all worry far too much about what everyone else is thinking and that creates a lot of anxiety for us all. If you feel chaotic when around others or in spaces that are crowded, just try to stick to your own small patch and what's going on within you. Create your own peaceful territory amongst the madness.

Summary

CREATE YOUR OWN SPACE.

Big, small, colourful, simple – make a physical space you can go for a spot of calm.

DECLUTTER.

Clear out the mess in your house and your head will follow!

TAKE CALM WITH YOU.

In 'un'calm places, breathe and remember calm is within you.

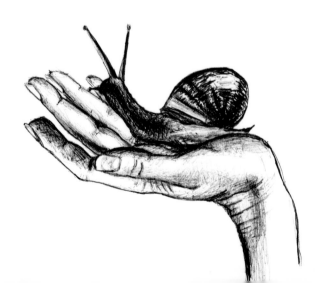

WHAT DOES A CALM ENVIRONMENT LOOK LIKE TO YOU?

Write one word or draw a picture here that sums it up.

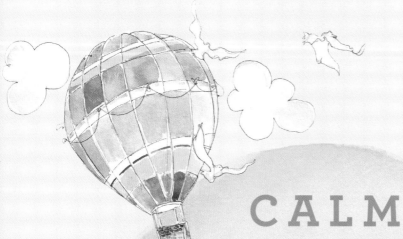

CALM
FUTURE
AND CALM
UNEXPECTED

Can you look into the future and feel safe? Can you peer out at the horizon and hope and believe that good will come? This will be much easier for some than others. My own trust and optimism has been diluted and compromised a little over the years as experience has stripped away layers of my confidence like peeling wallpaper, revealing a more delicate and exposed version of myself. I was possibly more robust in my teens and twenties as I had less experience of trauma and sorrow, and plain naivety added a lovely plump layer of armour.

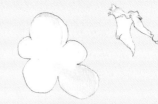

BE PREPARED

Most of us will know and understand that it is better to live in the NOW, grabbing hold of the moment and ekeing out what we can to make it really count. It's much easier said than done but there is a lot to be said for viewing what's around you in the moment, smelling the smells, listening to the sounds and feeling the emotions of what is NOW. This is a very powerful mindset that massively helps lead all of us back to calm. Extract the future from your now, this very millisecond you sit in, and you'll see that you're more than likely okay. If you are still in this moment and feeling sad, angry or overwhelmed, think again – are your present feelings about what is immediately happening to you now or is it due to what will or could happen in the future or what has happened in the past?

As much as we practise this theory and feel its benefits, in this day and age it is almost impossible NOT to look to what lies ahead. We have so much organising to do, what with work, social plans, family life and possible adventures that we need to go through the logistics of the future with a fine toothcomb. How easy is it to do this from a place of calm?

Some of us may actually feel calmer whilst preparing mentally for a situation that could unravel in the future rather than go with the flow of the unexpected. We can create our own safety blanket using preferred tricks that we have picked up along the way. Maybe a scary job interview is looming, but you know that preparation and study will be your tool of choice to calm your mind and defuse the buzz of energy you feel when you think to the future. Perhaps confrontation is on the cards and you feel that if you are more considered in your approach to this conversation there'll be less opportunity for clumsy mistakes and panic. I know that if I have a nerve-wracking job looming, by doing all the prep and studying I can on the situation I'll feel safer and calmer approaching the unknown. Stepping into new work arenas being ill-prepared instantly leads me to panic.

Having some positive thought and back-up plans in place will of course also be beneficial if you are waiting on the results of an exam or a health check, helping you to have a calmer acceptance of new information.

Preparing and being methodical in the present can help us to feel more in control and positive about the future, which should get us back to a calmer spot within.

FEAR OF WHAT-IFS

As I mentioned earlier in this book, in the Mind chapter, I have recently experienced the odd panic attack due to underlying stress and exhaustion that I hadn't taken proper notice of. For a while this experience gave birth to a new worry about driving at high speed. I used to cavort around the UK in my trusty Mini and even covered most of the USA in a yellow Mustang in the name of professional adventure, and not once did I feel anything other than sheer jubilation. This new fear was for a while relatively annoying, yet I knew it lived purely in a make-believe future. The fear was acutely attached to what might happen rather than what was presently happening. Due to some rather sturdy visualisations and a lot less stress in my life, I'm quite literally back

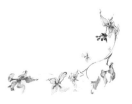

Even if we are currently feeling weak and scared there will have been moments where we have shown incredible amounts of strength. Drawing on these memories allows us to remember how resilient we can be when needed. Write a list of your own personal moments of hidden strength and remember your own ability and potential.

in the driving seat. In these moments I would try to get a hold on my breathing and slow it down, then visualise myself rooted deep into the ground. Suctioned to the core of the earth and all that is solid would stop my head from feeling so light it might float off my neck.

You may have a muscle memory anxiety about hypothetical future events, too. Maybe it's a situation that recurs, one that is drenched in fear and anxiety.

I think there are polarising reasons for why we are scared of certain what-ifs in the future. Either we are scared because these fears lie in the hands of fate and are unknown OR because we have suffered past trauma that stops us in our tracks and prevents us trying again.

TACKLING THE UNKNOWN

Let's start with the first reason; the delightful yet terrifying unknown. As small children we hurdle over 'firsts' with ease and determination. We take our first few steps on chubby feet and wobble and fall only to pop straight back up to try again. We may fall off our bikes several times after the removal of stabilisers but we will hop straight back on to give it another whirl. We talk to other kids we don't know with a lack of self-awareness or fear of rejection. It all feels like a liberating adventure rather than terrifying and debilitating. Somewhere along the line each of us loses this wild abandon somewhat and worry creeps into these cracks. Of course there will always be the odd incredible individual who remains maverick-like and all-round fearless but I can tell you now, I'm not one of them. I LOVE giving new things a go and continuously fidget until I've moved into new and challenging territory. I have changed career several times, left jobs I loved and tackled things I'm not naturally great at, all in the name of adventure and expansion. This does not mean I was lacking fear each time. Every step was taken with fear very firmly perched on my shoulders.

As we get older we hear more stories of people's mishaps and we are much more aware of others judging us. At times we stunt our own experiences out of fear of what others will say or how they will react, and this creates a lot of anxiety when trying something new. But I believe that we should all give our dreams and hopes a good go even if we feel this burden of judgment and fear. And I think there is a way of doing this from a place of calm rather than stress.

When I set out to write my first cookbook I was at times almost paralysed with worry about other people's perceptions of this venture. I was fresh out of a decade at Radio 1, where I used my music knowledge to get the job done, but cooking was not on the radar to the many that listened to me each day. Would people think I was a fraud? Would trained chefs laugh in my face and mock the book? Would anyone actually like what I had to offer?

The day before the book was released all excitement had been thwarted by a sense of imposter syndrome. Have you ever felt like this before? Like everyone else in your

When the unexpected leaps out of the dark it can whip us speedily away from calm. If you feel like you're trapped in a place of trauma can you start to work yourself back into the centre of these ripples, to your own calm? Try to work through some of these suggestions to see if they help.

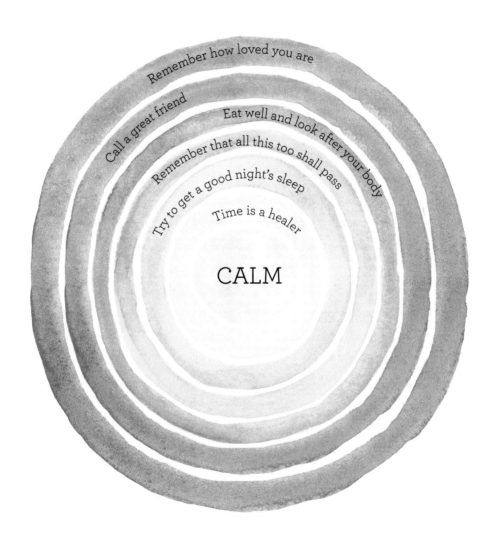

Remember how loved you are

Call a great friend

Eat well and look after your body

Remember that all this too shall pass

Try to get a good night's sleep

Time is a healer

CALM

field at work is acing it whilst you're merely blagging the hell out of it? I'm sure I can't be the only one out there who has been consumed by this suffocating feeling. Have you ever felt like someone may tap you on the arm at any minute and ask you to leave your place of work on the grounds that you are a fake? I'm pretty sure this feeling can happen to any of us, even those you may look up to in your own profession. There may be someone at work you admire greatly who you aspire to be like; I bet even they have felt like this on occasion. Even after 20 years, hundreds of live TV shows and countless interviews I still feel like I'm winging it at times. Even when I know exactly what I'm doing and feel pretty natural doing it my demons will pipe up and talk me down quite quickly. It can feel isolating as some folk out there are happy to display a startling confidence that acts as a veneer to cover their own fears and concerns. Luckily I have some pretty honest friends who work in the same game as me and are happy to admit their own mini freak-outs, which is instant solace for me.

Some individuals will sniff out this insecurity like a pig to truffles and enjoy feeding off the scraps of self-doubt that you have on display. Around the release of the cookbook there was one particular journalist who decided to grill me rather than interview me, with his sole mission seemingly being to put me down. As a sensitive person I don't always do well in these situations, so I felt even less confident about this book being seen by others. This 'first' was turning out to be a little more challenging than I had imagined. Luckily, once the book was released into the wild I had so much positive feedback, and I massively appreciate everyone who dipped into its pages and told me what they thought. I have also come to realise that the aforementioned journalist must view life in a very different way to me. This particular individual possibly doesn't want to see the good in others, or feels a sense of discomfort about his own achievements. I feel there must be a reason why he would come at something quite innocent from such an angle. I can only wish him well.

I think new endeavours are meant to be scary, but that fear shouldn't stop you doing what you truly want to do. We needn't worry about what others think when we want change in life. Change is nearly always traumatic as well as magical, as that is the paradoxical nature of its shift in energy. We must concentrate on getting ourselves through each scary moment in one piece and remember to enjoy life along the way. Luckily the experience of writing my first book turned into a very positive one and I sure as hell wasn't going to let one journalist spoil my mojo, so I have gone on to write several more. Each time I have had fear about people's thoughts and judgment, but I now try to view it all as an adventure rather than something to panic about. Ultimately, I'm glad I took the risk. Even if that cookbook hadn't been received well, I was putting something out there that I felt passionate about – it was always going to be worth a try and it was also very enjoyable as a challenge. Be risky, give newness a try, and focus on the positives in the future instead of the scary 'what if's.

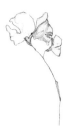

THE ORIGIN

If you feel scared about something on the horizon can you link it back to why? This often helps you gain clarity and perspective on the matter. Is it because you have failed previously in the same area? Or is it simply because it is 'the unknown'? Remember, life isn't repetitive. There is no set way in which your life will pan out and things can change in a heartbeat. If you're scared of making the same mistake, remember the outcome could be completely different to how it previously went. If you are scared because the unknown makes you feel unsafe, think back to a time in life when newness has been positive. There will be a few of these moments for everyone, I'm sure, even if it's a tiny moment that brought a new friend, job or adventure into focus. Recall those feelings and try to remember the same positivity can be injected into anything new that is on the horizon.

Do you ever feel it would be foolish to get excited about the future so instead you replace those feelings with dread or fear? Perhaps you've been hurt in the past and you don't trust the universe and all that lies ahead. I remember listening to an incredible podcast by Brené Brown, who is an analyst and inspirational talker I'm hugely fond of. She recalled an interview she had done for a study with a man whose wife had recently passed away. He said he was always scared to lean in to happiness and joy on the horizon in case the rug was pulled out from under his feet. Instead he tried to just sit in the middle of his emotions so as not to get hurt too badly. After his wife died he realised that living in such a way could never protect him from pain. He had wasted years like this and had still ended up without his wife. He was regretful that he hadn't leaned in to happiness and impending joy and that instead his fear had stunted his experience somewhat. So don't think it's foolish to look forward to events in the future. The universe isn't waiting to trip you up, nor will sitting stagnant somewhere in between it all protect you from stress or pain. If you feel excited, get excited, and enjoy every minute.

THE UNKNOWN IS POWERFUL

Above all, I think it's so important to remember that 'firsts' are really powerful because they help us to flow through life. Trying something new opens up space within us to learn more and see life more clearly. Each time we meet a new person or tackle a new challenge we are rewarded with some clarity and an expansive view of life. Even if the change or new circumstance feels traumatic or tough at the time, the lessons and increased vision will be 100 per cent there along the way. These opportunities allow us to think outside of the box and see new dimensions to life that we perhaps hadn't noticed before.

I've learned that when I get stuck in my ways and refuse change and newness I feel stagnant. I stunt my own learning and with passing time this becomes even more of an upheaval to change. We will have all felt stuck at some point in life, those moments where you want out or you feel an itch for change but don't act on it. We resist any change because it feels stressful and that is because we are scared. We are fearful of what might happen, even if we have an inkling that it could be for the best. I have discovered over the years that if I have had the idea or thought in the first place, it is probably a sign I should get a move on and give it a go. If I really need to, I will dig into my mental arsenal and pull out the most clichéd of all phrases, 'you only live once'. We all know how quickly time will pass and how years feel like they're slipping away in the blink of an eye, so why wait? I'm pretty sure most of us will get to a grand age with grey hair and a few stories to tell and we won't find ourselves wishing we DIDN'T give newness a go. I'm almost certain we won't feel regretful of the challenges we took on, even if we failed. We will only have regrets if we didn't try. Tackle newness and firsts with a sense of fun, mischief and adventure. Sure, fear and anxiety can come along for the ride if they insist, but they must take a back seat to allow us to really explore our full potential.

THE PAST AFFECTING THE FUTURE

So now on to that destructive anxiety that was born within the realms of the past. Here is a small example from my own life that doesn't cause me much worry or stress these days but has definitely got me into a weird habit that annoys the shit out of my mates. I will not pick up the phone. It is incredibly rare that I do and when those surprising moments arise my friends feel almost honoured that I dared to press 'ANSWER'. It all goes back to a few devastating phone calls I have received. Now when I hear that chirping of my phone my stomach flips and I assume it's someone calling to deliver bad news or tell me I've done something wrong. For me, it feels much less stressful and much calmer to just not pick it up. Annoying to many, I know, but hey, I'm a whiz on text! This is a tiny example of how our past can affect our general state of stress today, but it can of course get quite out of hand and be very debilitating. If we have experienced trauma how can we learn to trust in the unknown again? I believe it is possible, though, as many incredible people in my life have proved.

My dear friend Zephyr Wildman, who wrote the most glorious yoga section for my last book, *Happy*, has a back story steeped in pain and trauma but continues to live life in the most vivacious and positive way she can. Zephyr's husband died of cancer around seven years ago and she was left to raise their two small girls in the wake of this absurd trauma. I'm not sure how she climbed this huge mountain of pain and has come out stronger and even more incredible . . . but she has. Her girls are the most wonderfully smart and grounded young ladies and Zephyr has found love again. She married a brilliant man, Christian, who has taken on the role of dad to her children and has also given her the comfort and support she needs. She believed in love and also has a deep trust in life that has enabled her to fall into the arms of love without the constant worry or panic that it'll all be taken away from her again. She may be left with a morbid reality of how cruel life can be, but it hasn't stopped her finding the good stuff that she so wanted and deserved. This story is forever inspirational to me as it proves that we don't need to fear the future after experiencing loss or darkness in life. We can trust and overcome those fears and try again. It is possible to pick ourselves back up off the dusty floor of loss or failure and give it all another go.

I have been sacked from jobs, I've been dumped by many men, I've been mocked by strangers and I've missed personal goals by a long shot, but I haven't given up.

Sometimes we have to stop and pat ourselves on the back for simply carrying on. I'm so glad I didn't give up each time and lock myself away in a dark room full of books and biscuits (this is how I imagine I would live as a recluse), I have gone on to do jobs I love, find love and I keep getting more robust in my response to how others might judge me. There may be fear lurking around some subjects in my life and dark spots that need to be moved on but I have learned over the years not to let my back story define who I am today. Remembering that we don't have to BE our story allows us to let go of some of that tension and stress from who we 'think' we are. We assume we ARE all of our worries and fears. We ARE our failures and our weaknesses – but we really are NOT. Every single person out there, even if it doesn't look this way, has made mistakes, had shortcomings and struggles with something in life currently. Grasping hold of this concept allows us to step into new territory knowing that millions are going through the same thing and indeed have done so for thousands of years before us.

There will be some trauma in life that seems immovable. Horror stories that have a cinematic quality and won't leave your mind. These stubborn creases in life may at times need ironing out with the help of others. Maybe you have a dear friend who knows you inside out, who can help you see the light again. If not, maybe some professional trauma counselling is the one for you. No one should have to live in fear of the past or indeed the future due to historical events. Everyone has the right to start over.

Sometimes we need permission from another to let go of old habits and patterns caused by an event in the past. Sometimes we need that gentle reminder that we don't have to be our back story. We can sit calmly in the NOW, knowing that all that has happened can have an impact but doesn't define us.

THE PAST

All of us fear things in the future due to our past. It's a work in progress to not let things that have previously occurred affect us now but it is possible. The first step is recognising the memories that determine portions of our lives now. On the timeline below fill in the years that are relevant to you and write down the past events that have affected how you live today. In the boxes closer to 'Today' write the occasions and worries that you know are affected by these past events.

TODAY

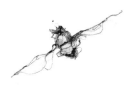
IMAGINING THE FUTURE

When I'm worried about something that's coming up, I like to run through some visualisations to help me feel calmer, picturing situations as I want them to happen and imagining the feeling and emotions that could arrive in these moments. Of course, we never know what life might throw our way, but running through scenarios and the way we can react to them gives us the confidence to know that we can get through them should they arise.

Visualising and dreaming what we want to happen can also be a lot of fun. If it's all coming from a positive place there is no harm in visualising those wonderful situations that you dream will come into fruition. We must expect the odd plot twist but if we are open to change and opportunity, even if things don't pan out exactly as we had imagined, at least we know we are being sent off in another direction that could be equally as exciting or a good learning curve.

I have always strongly visualised being a mother. I have pictured children in my story from the get go and was lucky enough to have this dream come true. My plot twist was also receiving step-children along the way. I had never imagined or given much thought to this possibility but I went with this new tangent and love my new role as a step-mother alongside being a mum to my own kids. Motherhood didn't end up being exactly as I had imagined and visualised, and I knew from this point onwards having my own kids alongside my step-children would mean a lot of work and organisation – but that didn't matter to me at all and now I can't imagine my life any other way. Accepting there may well be varying outcomes to our dreams and hopes stops us from getting too freaked out about new tangents. It also leaves room to view clearly what we can gain from unexpected happenings. Lessons learned, love in unexpected forms, new ideas and thoughts on life; it's all up for grabs if we aren't too set in our ways as to how our life should pan out.

FINDING CALM IN THE UNEXPECTED

So how do we keep calm in sight when we feel completely derailed in life? When the unexpected is thrown in our face at great speed and we are blind to the good and inner calm? There have been a few moments in my own life where nothing made sense. Out of the blue came unwanted situations that seemed to serve no use at the time. I couldn't see the lessons that could be learned or that any expansion was possible at all, and this makes for a very discombobulated existence. In these moments I think time is the greatest comfort to lock sight on. On occasion it can be the only thing you can grab hold of out of desperation; everything else feels far too slippery and uncertain, but the ticking of the clock is a guarantee. It's a tiny comfort to sink into to help us on the way back to calm. Most situations will have an expiry date – bad times end, clarity will be gained and lessons will fall into place. As ghastly as my own traumas may have been for me, I am able to see the positives that felt invisible at the time. Next time I am derailed in life, I am hoping that instead of fear and panic I am able to integrate a little more calm into proceedings knowing that the situation will pass, as it has before; that I will expand mentally and emotionally along the way; and that these stories and moments do not define me. I'm not sure anyone out there has completely nailed this one but I think we all get slightly better at it as we gain more experience.

Another personal mantra I try to bring into focus is 'does this really matter?'. Sometimes tough moments will seem very dramatic and chaotic but they can actually be solved or ironed out with a little thought and a calm approach. If it's a situation that we know deep down has a minimal aftermath, we know down the line this moment will be forgotten altogether. We may still learn the odd lesson, but the impact of these moments are tiny bumps in the road rather than gaping canyons. If I'm running late for something I am prone to getting quite red-faced and stressed as I don't want to let people down or seem rude. I have to navigate back to the thought that, within the bigger picture, this moment won't have any catastrophic outcome. If someone is upset by my tardiness I will apologise and it is then up to them as to how long they hold on to that annoyance.

If my kids don't eat their dinner I start to feel tense and anxious as I feel as if I have failed as a mother. I panic that I have not instilled the necessary discipline or courage in them to try new foods and will therefore beat myself up about it constantly. Again, if I pull focus and remember that it really doesn't matter and that they will more than likely eat better next week, I can let go of that anxiety. It doesn't serve any purpose. It is not teaching me any lessons, my kids don't need me acting from an uptight place and it certainly won't change the problem at hand. These small stresses in life are unfortunate but we mustn't lose sight of their size; we mustn't blow them up and inflate their importance, as that stress can far too quickly become our default setting in life and we then get into a state when something doesn't go our way. This sort of stress might not seem worthy of discussion but I think a lot of us are drowning in the minor problems in life and actually this underlying stress is causing many mental and physical problems. For me it may lead to a headache, backache or a dysfunctional digestive system. For you it may be backache, insomnia or a skin problem. This stress could be taking its toll on a relationship or stopping you from simply having fun. This lethargic, overflowing stress about the mundane things in life has to have an outlet, and more often than not it's a physical one. The banal underlying stress triggers so many other unwanted and undesirable problems in life that we have to work hard to observe it and stop these dirty habits in their tracks. It's simply not worth it.

Then come the life explosions that really do seem to matter. The big ones: loved ones getting sick or when we are left abandoned in life or perhaps have our own health issues. Journeying through moments like this can feel like an arduous and impossible trek with no end in sight. This is when we have to lean on others. This is when that robust web of friendships needs to be tested out. Never be afraid to lean on friends – and family – they can often be the ultimate stress-relievers.

If the tough situation you are enduring feels isolating and you're not sure that any of your loved ones will offer the needed support and empathy, look to local support. Is there a group near you that could help you feel understood? Is there an NHS-supported counselling service to lend a comforting ear? Or perhaps you could just do something new in your day where you can give yourself a little escapism from the heavy situation that you're living through. Feeling supported and heard in these moments is unbelievably important, because adding loneliness and isolation to the already overflowing plate of shit is not what we need.

In these heavy times, lessons will feel unwanted and harder to swallow but they might just help you see a small flicker of light somewhere down the line. Maybe you'll be spun off in a new life direction once you've managed to get yourself out of the darkness. Maybe you'll view life in a completely different way. Maybe you'll feel everything more intensely and seek out the deep and meaningful in life in ways you hadn't before. I think trauma can chuck in some interesting options at times. They might not be a magic cure to the pain and suffering but they may help you get through it. If panic feels like your default setting due to trauma, seek support and be kind and gentle with yourself. Don't feel guilty for making these things a priority. We need self-love and self-care in tough times so that we can get through these treacherous passages in one piece.

EXPECT THE UNEXPECTED (AND ENJOY IT!)

As I mentioned earlier, from experience, I think the worst road to take is one that's static. If we don't at least open our eyes to change and a potential solution we stand little chance of moving fluidly through stress-fuelled periods. If we expect change to spring out of the abyss we are more than likely to end up stuck in quicksand with no way out. It is surprising how much strength we have hidden within, and these super powers seem to be tightly bound with calm. Think back to that light springing out of your sternum. We all have this strength within us, it's not an exclusive attribute for a chosen few. If we open our hearts and dig deep we will have this burning ember waiting to be reignited and put to use. This strength can at times have the power to combat fear and panic and can make you feel slightly more in control, or at least feel okay in the chaos. Surrendering to panic will rarely do much good. We will spin further out of control and start to believe that our own well of calm has run dry for good. Remember your own strength and recall times when you have put it to good use. There will be moments threaded through your life that you can look back on and celebrate. These moments don't have to define who we are but they can certainly remind us of what we are all personally capable of.

THE (SOMETIMES) BUMPY ROAD BACK TO CALM

This doesn't mean that we have to put on a perpetually brave face or cover up what we are really feeling, in fact it's quite the opposite. This inner strength can enable us to let those emotions flow naturally as they come and go, but with a knowledge that they are not permanent. We can let fear flow through our veins, we can allow anxiety to wash over our clammy skin and we can give anger a moment to explode out of every pore. I have personally found that suppressing emotions and feelings just means we hold it back in a giant dam, only to be released at a later and possibly inconvenient date. We should never feel scared to feel the emotions bubbling away or think we have to validate what they mean. We all have the right to feel exactly what seems appropriate – as long as we don't hold on to these feelings for dear life and make them permanent friends. We must all experience those feelings and express them accordingly but we must not get stuck. Pitching up camp in limbo land is excruciating for all those involved. It may seem like a calmer dwelling but that's only because it often disguises itself as a safe place to stop. This limbo land may display comfort and momentary ease but it will more than likely make any change in the future that bit tougher. If we are feeling stressed and a long way from calm we have to try to look at ways in which we can move forward. This doesn't mean moving away from or abandoning obstacles in life, it simply means to seek out support, a change or a solution. Perhaps sometimes we have to resort to boring old practicality and making considered pragmatic moves in the direction of change. There may not seem like many available options at times but small tweaks are just as important as great leaps. I'm pretty sure we will have all been in destructive relationships or at least know others who have been; it is so easy to stay put and feel like we should just float in limbo until we are forced to make changes or decisions. Surely that limbo is easier and calmer than making any significant change? Well, unfortunately it's not. As traumatic and sometimes wrong as it may feel, change is imperative to get us out of stagnant situations and for us to continue growing and feeling good. Although there may be volcanic trauma at first this will eventually lead to a solid calm that we can relax into. The path back to calm isn't always an easy ride but if we make changes to uncomfortable or stressful circumstances we're one step closer.

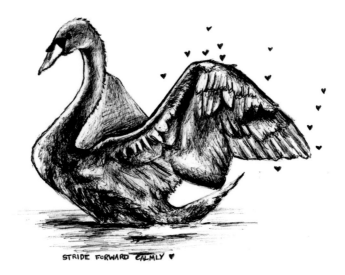

STRIDE FORWARD CALMLY ♥

Summary

HARNESS YOUR INNER CHILD.

When you're nervous about the unknown, remember how many 'firsts' you've conquered in your life. You've got this!

LOOK FORWARD.

Don't let the past affect your present – or your future. Leave it where it belongs.

EXPECT THE UNEXPECTED . . .

. . . And revel in the wonders it can bring!

WHAT DOES A CALM FUTURE LOOK LIKE TO YOU?

Write one word, or draw a picture here that sums it up?

CALM AND THE OUTSIDE WORLD

The world seems busier than ever, faster than ever, and most definitely more stressed than ever. Is this a reality or just what we are seeing because we can so easily tap into everyone else's lives whenever we desire it? A 24/7 vision of not only our own chaos staring back at us, but everyone else's too! This constant download of information about other members of our families, communities and corners of the planet makes us feel like everything is so very busy. We are constantly observing, judging, comparing and trying to make sense of so much information. Rather than just viewing life through one set of eyes, we are viewing life on our phones, computers and TVs, so it's a constant information overload.

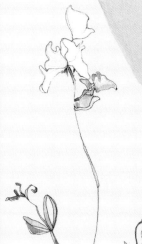
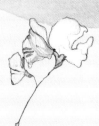
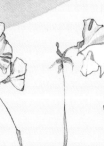
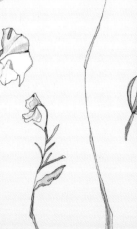

LOOKING AROUND US

Along with this daily overstimulation we are also bombarded with options. This is so new to the human race and perhaps at its pinnacle right now. We have hundreds of TV channels, social media outlets, shops, people, cuisines, apps, ways to travel, ways to date and myriad jobs that we can do, so it's no wonder we are seemingly more confused than ever. With so much choice, we spread ourselves thinly rather than concentrating on fewer things to the best of our ability. We are mostly a culture of overstimulated, confused worriers. The anxiety is everywhere, alongside the options, and it's hard not to feel this way with so much activity and information whizzing in and out of our lives. It seems our heads are the busiest part of it all, not necessarily just the world around us.

Some mornings I will peel back the curtains and be swarmed with a feeling of excitement and endless opportunity. There seems to be a world of adventure to be explored: new people to meet, new places to go and new lessons to be learned. I have a dawning of subconscious realisation that I am part of this worldwide energy. A tiny cog that plays a part in it all. Then I gain perspective and I understand my actual size. I am tiny yet vital in the vastness of constant movement across the planet. My world and all of its drama, excitement and worry is just a speck in this intricate picture that makes up this spinning ball of our planet out in space. I sink into this harmony and calm floods my day and all that stands in my way. I'm sure we have all experienced this glorious feeling at times and how the magic of the outside world can offer up opportunity and allows us to dream and create.

On other days, that morning visual of everyone else going about their business reminds me of the sheer chaos on planet Earth and it makes me panic about my place in it all. On those heavier days where I feel overwhelmed, it's as if I can sense the pain of every suffering being out there. I become acutely aware of the struggles and injustice that flows from all corners of the planet and am struck by the impossible task of making it all okay, or at the very least making sense of it all. In this day and age where we all move so fast and consume so much, we often forget how much information we are all taking on board every single second of the day. It's not just the walk to work or the school gates in the morning, it's the onslaught of information pouring through the bright lights of our smartphones and every picture leaping from the pages of papers and magazines in the shops that we pass. It's every word of gossip spoken and every text message and email gobbled down. It may feel normal to us but we are one of the first few generations experiencing this level and brevity of noise and information. Images, news and ideas are now quicker, exaggerated and feel almost like a 'must' if we are to keep up with the velocity in which we live.

STEP AWAY FROM THE PHONE

A gradual change has taken place in many parts of the world over the last ten or so years, where, as a race, our thumbs have become more agile, our necks have begun to slant downwards and our vision is blinkered. PHONES. In the western world, we are mostly all guilty of this but are any of us concerned enough to do anything about it?

Can we even see how our inner calm is being compromised by this constant action? In this day and age it would be pretty impossible to live without a phone, but how much do we let it run the show and how aware are we of our attachment to it? I am as guilty as anyone else with this; I find the temptation to check emails whilst I'm out and about, or flick through Instagram when I'm procrastinating, near impossible to ignore. It's so ingrained in my day that I sometimes find myself mindlessly on my phone without thought or concern. How much am I missing out on what is going on around me by using this tactic of distraction? Probably quite a lot. In my teens I would catch the train to London a lot. This was a time before mobile phones were commonplace and certainly before social media and apps. My phone would be firmly tucked into a pocket of my rucksack as I would only need TO locate it if I had to call someone or check the time. Now if I'm on the train or even just walking down the road, 80 per cent of people are completely unaware of what is going on around them as their necks are craned down in the direction of their screens. AND I'm usually one of them. I'm trying hard to break this habit as I know I am missing out on a possibly calm scene or even just the mental space for new ideas and thoughts. Social media and the internet are obviously gorgeous ways to connect with friends on other sides of the planet, as well as catch up on news and information about things we might otherwise miss out on, but whilst doing this, we are trading the simple and calm in life for it. We have swapped observing our surroundings and the people around us for the far away and distant. It's a strange swap when you break it down; the more we are on our phones the more we feel the need to be abreast of everything that is going on around us. The need to feed this habit grows the more we do it and we start to feel edgy without it.

It's like any habit: we forget the negative impact and go with the initial desire.

So back to when I was 18, on the train in London and have forgotten my book. I might people-watch, let my brain wander and create stories about other people in the carriage. I might catch the eye of someone else and smile. I might notice an interesting house outside the train. I'm pretty certain that a lot more people would meet new people, start conversations, perhaps even flirt when out and about back then, because we would actually notice those around us. Phones stop us from connecting with the outside world in a way which was seen as natural and normal 15 years ago. I endeavour to open my eyes and all other senses to what's happening around me at least once a day. That feels much more calming and expansive to me than being a slave to my phone and its many apps. Perhaps try it too? Maybe on your way to work or while walking today, put your phone in your pocket and look around you properly. Maybe you'll smile at someone, maybe you'll offer to help someone struggling to get a buggy up a flight of stairs, maybe you'll spot a beautiful tree. Open up your senses and be in your true surroundings. The more we do this the more inner calm we'll be able to access. I'm sure as hell going to give it a good try!

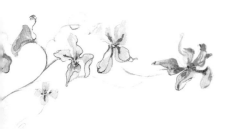

HOW TO DEAL WITH THE ONSLAUGHT OF MEDIA

There seems to be little protection against this onslaught of stimulation because we are beginning to think this is a normal way to live. There is no filter or remedy to the invasion of data we try to pack into our overflowing minds. There may be suggestions and a more holistic approach available if we are that way inclined, but these methods of detoxing the mind are still seen as perhaps a luxury or an out-of-the-box choice rather than a necessity.

This has been a gradual realisation for me and I have noticed my instincts and choices have started to go against the grain somewhat. I used to be able to binge-watch any TV show; I would consume programmes of a stressful nature, watch the odd bit of cinematic violence and wasn't bothered by the high-octane action threaded through storylines. Over the last few years, in which I have begun to dig deeper and explore varying avenues of self-care, I've realised that I cannot continue with this habit. I can only watch shows that are of a true nature, displaying biopic stories from which I can learn, or feel-good comedy and fiction. Anything else leaves me wired and slightly exhausted. I know this may sound dramatic but I think now having a greater understanding of how I work has left me needing to switch off in my downtime instead of introducing unnecessary stress, even if it does live within the confines of a TV screen.

I'm making more conscious decisions around what I fill my brain with. After having experienced the unwanted and dramatic at times in my own life I understand how out of control we can all feel, and this has led me to pay more attention as to how I consume information around me and how much I choose to download mentally. My decision always starts with the question, 'will this take me to a place of calm?' We can't ignore what is going on around us at home, locally or worldwide but we do have a choice as to how much we take on board, especially in a fictional sense.

We are all constantly bombarded with news. It is hard to avoid because our phones, TVs, radios and the papers shout about the latest tragedy or sorrow. Although we cannot live in a bubble where we have no clue as to what is going on outside of our own homes, I do think we have to be sensitive as to how and when we take this information on board. Maybe reading the papers in the morning makes you feel informed and stable at the start of your day, and if that's the case, carry on as you are. Perhaps for some of you it is hard to take on any more negativity as you feel you're dealing with enough in your own life. I oscillate between the two; sometimes I read about tragedy and disaster and the stories fill me with compassion and empathy. I might feel powered up by a story I've read and a yearning to help others. On tougher days, personally I may feel I can't take on any more sorrow. I have nothing to give as I haven't sorted out my own array of problems, so I leave those stories until I can react in a calmer and possibly more helpful manner. On certain days where I've felt far from buoyant I won't put on the news in the evening, as the constant rolling fear and sadness that flies out of our screens feels too much to take on before I go to bed. Instead I will look through websites the next morning when I know I can keep on top of world news in a more controlled way.

There is no wrong or right – I think you just have to know your own personal limits and expectations. Taking on every single bit of information and negativity doesn't

make you a better person, as some seem to believe. I believe what is most important is how compassionate you are towards those you are reading about or how proactive you are towards subjects that ignite a flame within. Knowing everything all of the time doesn't make the world a better place or inflate your intellectual status to outshine others. If you can happily take on board a lot of outside drama and stress without it having much effect on your own life, then go with it, but if you know it takes its toll, you have every right to seek out the stories that make you feel uplifted instead. As well as feeling deep compassion for anyone out there suffering, as well as doing some much-loved charity work for those I feel I can help, I personally need to find that balance of negative and positive in the world. If I feel I have digested both in equal measure I feel calmer and more balanced and will hopefully be of more use in any way I can.

Being sucked into the storm of negativity that is whirling around out there is only helpful if you're willing to make a change in some way – perhaps a small personal change you believe will have a ripple effect or, if you can, big social changes that you believe in. I think ranting and shouting rarely does much good as it only ignites more fury. If you believe that only awful things occur on planet Earth, that's all you'll ever see. I believe there are equal measures of both out there, it's just unfortunate that the negative stories gain a lot more traction. Very rarely will a story be uplifting or enlightening, so balancing out this information with stuff that makes you feel good is vital to help you remember that hope and positivity have a place on Earth, too.

Some believe that evil is on the rise and that more people are thinking selfishly and dangerously, as we are constantly shown images and told stories where injustice is rife and pain rules. Although it is true that this chaos exists and can be very extreme at times, we have to remember that there has to be a 50/50 balance to align with nature and how the world has always worked. I think we just hear about the negative a lot more these days and have 24/7 access to it. There has always been conflict, war and disagreement and probably always will be – these days we just have many more channels through which to receive news of this daily trauma.

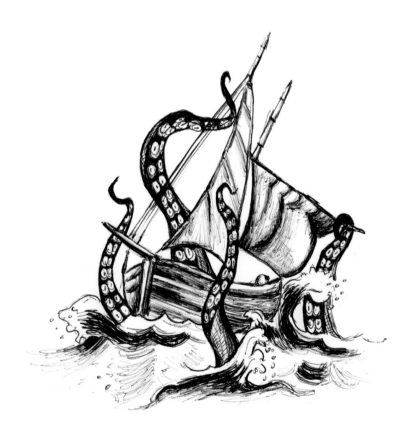

Taking on board what is depicted in the media is almost a given in this day and age. It's pretty impossible to ignore it, but we do have a certain control over how much we consume. Write in the newspaper on the left-hand side how much news, gossip and social media you think you mentally download each day, and see if you could balance it out with any of the suggestions on the right-hand page.

THE GOOD NEWS

Read a feel-good book

Send a friend a letter.
Oh how I love snail mail

LISTEN TO MUSIC
THAT MAKES
YOU FEEL ALIVE

Research a subject online
that you're interested in

Look at old photos
that make you feel lovely

DOWNLOAD AN
INTERESTING PODCAST

REJECT NEGATIVITY

Does this negativity change how we talk to others around us, does it fill us with fear so that we feel stilted in life, or does it simply add to the anger of a previous personal situation? I think at times we don't even see how much this adds to our personal load until we take a look at how much we are consuming digitally and globally, daily. If your calm is being stripped away by overconsumption, take a look at how much you are viewing each day and how you choose to download what is going on around you.

It's the same with outside gossip, whether in magazines or in your own circle. How much does negative conversation affect you deep down? How much salacious chat do you digest and how much of it lives on in your physical being? I know that if I've been tempted by gossip, either about somebody close to me or not, I feel physically grim and slightly grubby. As tantalising as gossip may seem, it never quite fills the hole that your own sense of lacking something has left. Judging others and having our say on how other people live their lives doesn't mitigate our own problems. After these empty conversations shut down we are invariably left feeling worse than before.

Do you have a mate who only deals in gossip? Perhaps their everyday vernacular is tinged with a spiky hunger to view and mock others? If that friend's words seem to stick to you like glue and feel like they're dragging you far from your own personal calm, maybe it's time to switch things up. Is there a chance you could try to change their point of view? Suggest how they could see things from a different angle or get off the subject of others for a while? If negative chat leaves you feeling like you need a good shower, shake off those unwanted words and stories and extract yourself from the circle of gossip you're in.

HOW WE VIEW OTHERS

The way in which we digest gossip online has also started to be viewed as the 'norm'. We are far too used to seeing women pitted against each other, labelled with tags and descriptions that only tell a tiny percentage of their story. It is not shocking for us to view tales of female weight loss and style 'wrongs' glaring back at us from magazines. On the front pages we constantly see women celebrated for the wrong things and judged for the ridiculous. This takes me far from my place of calm. Sure, women can lose weight if they choose. They can also adorn themselves with dreamy clothes and do what they like with make-up and hair styles, but that doesn't mean that those are the only subjects worth discussing. I love looking at women's fashion and style but surely it shouldn't be used as a measure to gauge other women's worth and position in the world. How are we, as a society, supposed to consume this sort of information about others and then feel okay ourselves? If it is so readily acceptable to make stark assumptions about women we don't really know, how are young women supposed to celebrate themselves and their own quirks? I believe the ways in which females are depicted in the media and online can be very damaging for us all, but especially for the younger generation who are navigating through the rough terrain of teenhood with an even louder volume of self-awareness thrown into the mix. There have been a couple of occasions where I myself have been subject to this sort of objectifying. Just after I had given birth to my daughter Honey I was photographed in a bikini on holiday with my family. There I was, with my postnatal doughy belly out and my milky breastfeeding bulging boobs desperately trying to escape my bikini top. Magazines printed these pictures for all to see with peculiar text suggesting it was a relief to see a mum looking out of shape. Firstly, what do you expect? Only three months before I had pushed an eight-pounder out of my lady parts and was at this point keeping said gorgeous baby alive solely with my milk! Secondly, why is it a relief? Why can't we all just be the shape and size we are without constant comparison and judgment? If someone has just had a baby, let that be that. If someone loves to work out every day and has abs of steel, let them be that. It seems absurd for us all to need constant markers of where we fit in to everything in such an aesthetic manner.

When I was a teenager I didn't have this issue to battle with as I had a brick-like mobile phone that could only call people. Social media hadn't been dreamt up and magazines weren't quite so prolific in their subject matter. I could ramble on through my teen years, stumbling over the speed bumps of first break-ups, periods and acne without much pressure. I may have still felt completely freaked out at each learning curve but I had no idea about how the masses were judging the situations that young women face. I had little comparison other than whispers from my friend Becky, who has an older sister. This is how we digested new information and viewed other girls – through the snippets of advice and news we may have siphoned from a friend's older sibling. All pretty harmless and, looking back, pretty hysterical. I dread to think how I would have coped living a double life on social media at that age. I can only just about deal with it at the age of 36.

Now there seems to be an unspoken rule book of how women should be, to avoid being ripped apart by others. Even if we aren't consuming this information in a literal sense, some of it will seep in by osmosis to us all. Even if we refuse to look on social

Gossip is so seductive and near impossible to avoid at times. We get such a high and instant rush from it as we lose our footing from calm and forget that the oppositeside of the high is waiting imminently on the other side. Write down who you regularly gossip about and notice how it makes you really feel. Do you feel an initial sugar rush high from it, but come crashing down on the other side? Or do you feel like you need a good bath when the rant is over? Mark on the graph where the gossip takes you.

I gossip about ....

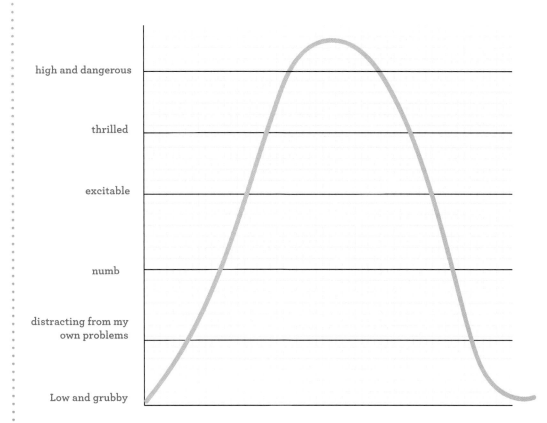

high and dangerous

thrilled

excitable

numb

distracting from my
own problems

Low and grubby

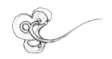

media or don't buy into an editorial portrayal of the female form, we are aware of the images of supposed extreme perfection. We also see them so regularly that we forget they're extreme and not regular or relatable to the masses at all. This can be the biggest confidence killer and can be fairly stressful for a lot of us ladies out there.

I'm pretty sure each one of us will at some point have thought obsessively about a body part we hate. Mine...? There are a few. A large forehead (which I cover with face-framing hair – you will NEVER see me with my hair worn back) and broad shoulders to start with. Why would I have conjured up the idea that these body parts were 'wrong'? No other person in my life has ever mentioned either of these body insecurities to me but because I go on social media, because I look in magazines, I know that the 'ideal' women shown do not have either of these attributes. I'm also not particularly fond of my nose as it seems too pointy and prominent on my face. I've not seen many females in editorial images or in Disney films with anything other than a cute button snout, so mine seems a little . . . well, 'wrong'. I hate to use that word as I'm all for quirks and celebrating our uniqueness but I'd be lying to you if I said I didn't have negative thoughts about this at times. Mostly, though, I'm grateful. At this age I can route back to basics and strip away the reflex comparisons and give thanks for all my quirks. In fact, on a good day, I'll really enjoy my characterful nose and dinner plate forehead.

These thoughts are only spurred on by comparison, though, as that's the template we all seem to work from these days. Compare and despair. I'm very grateful I have a working and healthy body, so none of these annoyances are particularly debilitating in life – my nose is pretty good at keeping me alive, with its air-inhaling nostrils, and my broad shoulders help me with my love of yoga, so there are many positives to outweigh the negatives. I'm simply being as honest as I can to show you how we are all affected by what we see daily. I'm also pretty sure all of us will have made sweeping statements about a celebrity in a magazine, stating we don't like their clothes or hair. I most definitely have and it never feels good. Who cares what I think or have to say about that celebrity? At the time that individual felt great in their clothes and also has a whole huge life beyond that one tiny photo.

I feel so far from calm when I pay attention to this glaring issue that women have to face, but I know the only thing I can do is scramble back to my place of calm, remembering all the wonderful beliefs I personally have about women. If we can look past the obsession of aesthetic and generalising specifications aimed at women, we can celebrate and illuminate a plethora of inspirational, kick-ass, game-changing qualities that all of us possess. It doesn't matter if we feel different to what we see out there, and it shouldn't have any bearing on how we think about any other females. We can go about our business in our own way, viewing other women in our lives with compassion, empathy and an open heart. We all feel insecure, vulnerable and scared at some point and there are no exceptions to this story. We can still gorge on magazines, buy all the delicious clothes on offer, wear as much or as little make-up as we choose to, we can be as voluptuous and beautiful or slight and delicate as we naturally are or choose to be. None of this matters to anyone else and nor should those decisions made be open for judgment by others. Knowing that allows us all to digest as much online or editorial gumpf as we desire but from a more grounded, balanced and calm place.

We can also be inspired by these outlets, though, which is the great part! We can see someone who is achieving their goals and chooses to calmly feel inspired rather than envious. We can view another life and think that person seems happy then calmly endeavour to feel that happiness in our own way. As long we all remember that a lot of what we are viewing is tinged with fantasy and assumption, we can calmly take on board what we see and can feel inspired rather than lacking.

BE AT PEACE WITH WHO YOU ARE

If you feel judged by others and that pressure is causing you undue stress, just remember one thing; when others openly judge you it says far more about THEM than it does you. Knowing this will always whisk you back towards your place of calm, because realising that the opinions of others are purely based on THEM and what THEY'RE lacking, allows you to carry on as you were.

We don't have to fit in, be the same or conform to social-media-driven conditions either. We just need to feel calm doing things our own way – calm leads to confidence. It allows us to wear our own colours with a bold smile on our face. It gives us the ability to enjoy feeling different. Yet being different in any way can instantly lead to an acute panic because we can feel alienated or alone. The word 'different' shouldn't even make sense in this situation as we obviously all differ in every way. That's the magic of being a human, no? We each have a unique look, thought process, experience of life and way of seeing things. We may find comfort in a community or group but really we are all very different from each other – magical friendship and unions are created based

We all feel judged in one way or another by other people, but more often than not that judgment is only coming from ourselves. Others may highlight our weaknesses but really we are the ones giving ourselves a hard time. Give yourself a pat on the back: write down everything you've done, however small, that you're proud of below.

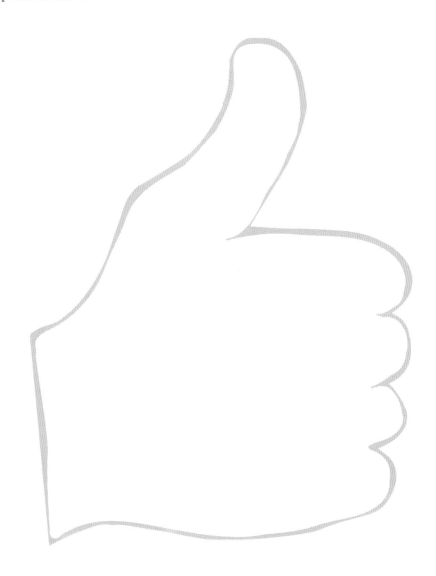

on connections and not similarity. There is no 'same'.

An illusion has been created over the years of what it takes to be a man or a woman, but that is just a one-dimensional idea, it's not the truth of the matter. There is no real conforming because there is no real template as to how, for example, a woman should be. Be YOU and be free in this thought. Lose the stress of trying to be the female you think you should be and feel calm being the female that you ARE. Be a maverick, be an anomaly, go against the grain and feel okay doing it.

At times I can do this with ease and aplomb, loving every second of walking in my own lane. Other times I feel like I'm walking on melting ice yet with subzero waters below. Getting back to your own calm and knowing it is okay to do as you please may take time but it is possible. You don't have to block out what the rest of the world is up to; you can take it on board then charge forward knowing your way is equally as valid as anyone else's. It takes guts and an open heart and most definitely a huge slice of calm.

OVERSHARING

The other side of the coin to 'how much we digest' is how much we choose to 'share'. We are apparently the generation of oversharers, as again we have become accustomed to letting the world see us from many angles. In comparison to two decades ago, this seems very true. When I was growing up I would perhaps take two disposable cameras away on holiday with me or maybe a cheap digital camera and take up to 50 snaps of my trip. This seemed sufficient for a good reminisce on my return. These days we probably take half of that in a single day when we are just at home. Our phones are usually permanently glued to our hands, snapping away at any given moment, whether it contains any magic or not. Back then I would take my camera down to my local high street to get the 50 pictures developed and show them to my best mate, who was seemingly not that bothered by the incredible sunset I had witnessed on night two of my break. (Aren't other people's holiday's photos the most boring thing on Earth?!) These days we upload any number of these photos to Instagram, Twitter or Facebook for our friends to swipe by and comment on if they choose. Today it is almost odd to not know where one of your friends might be in the world, as they are always contactable and more than likely viewable too. I remember when I was 15, bumping into one of my best mates in Mallorca as neither of us had any idea we would both be on our family holidays in the same week. This would never happen these days as we always know where everyone is.

This oversharing and knowing everyone's business has become the norm but it might be playing havoc with how we live our lives and how much we are losing a grip on calm. I definitely feel like I have to email people back instantly or text a response as otherwise someone might assume something has happened to me. This pressure is not calming in any way, shape or form. I turned my phone off for one day last week and many of my mates were wondering why the hell I wasn't texting back – 15 years ago I might not hear from a close friend in two weeks as it would involve a pay phone or snatched moment on the house phone, but this didn't dilute friendships or stop the flow of chat at all. So why are we so scared to be uncontactable? Perhaps we fear we may miss out on something great then have to see it on Facebook later? Perhaps we

What moments in your life have felt completely magical and full of love?

feel we may lose a grip on the news and what is going on around us and fall behind? Maybe we feel if we don't share online we'll become unpopular or less desirable as a friend. Of course none of these things will happen but the speed of today's communication and ability to reach one another gives us an illusion of otherwise.

Obviously being able to Google information quickly is a wonder and speaking to a friend on FaceTime who lives thousands of miles away is a gift, so there are some heavenly spots within this fast-paced way of living. But we need to remember that it's not the only way and it's not vital all of the time. If we give ourselves breaks from it all and remember that many generations before us lived perfectly well without this constant communication, we can remove some of the stress and just enjoy the handy/fun parts. I cannot stand the online catchphrase 'photo or it didn't happen'. Not only have its school-yard connotations got an annoying sing-song ring but it also speaks volumes about how we view life. Private, golden magic moments seemingly can't breathe or exist unless they are shared with hundreds of others. This cannot be true and I'll tell you why.

Close your eyes now and grab hold of a moment that for you felt like the clock stopped ticking. A moment where you felt 100 per cent alive and free and knew that moment counted for something. It contained magic and a warmth that is now unfathomable. I have a handful of these moments that I can pull out of my memory bank whenever I please and feel forever grateful of this. Holding my two babies in my trembling arms seconds after they had entered the world. Sitting on the edge of a pool drinking a beer in Mexico as birds sang above my head and my skin felt warm from the afterglow of a sunny day. Walking away from a bar in Ibiza knowing I had met someone very special (I'm now married to him). These moments are heavily stitched into my story and have a luminous quality about them in my mind. None of these moments were 'shared' in a photo. No one else saw them, felt them or knew about them. They are for me to unlock when I need to. I can access any one of these dreamlike scenes on down days and know that more magic is out there waiting to be captured.

Sharing online is a lot of fun and can be interesting and inspiring but we mustn't forget to grab hold of life without our phones in hand so we can drink down these moments fully, experiencing them for what they are. These moments bring the calm and get you back to what you know you love and believe.

FINDING A WAY OUT OF THE NOISE

So how can we block out this constant noise around us? We can't fully and most of us don't want to either. It's more about quality control and our perception of what is going on around us. That's how we can regain any calm in moments of chaos. I think working out what makes you feel good, inspired (even if that is a little fired up) and open, against what makes you feel empty, scared and angry, is the first port of call. Once you sit and view these daily joys and anxieties you can start to monitor how you take in this information. For example, there was a time when I used to always flick through Instagram before I went to bed. I knew what every one of my friends was up to, what Katy Perry had eaten for lunch and what shoes I really now lusted after. None of this information was conducive to a good night's sleep and it also made me feel slightly wired. I would feel my muscles tense, my brain cogs whirring and then the compare and despair would start.

This would rumble on until I fell into a broken and bumpy night's sleep. I recognised this, after possibly too big a chunk of time, and decided this weird pre-sleep ritual had to go. Reading a good book in the bath is working out as a much better option for me these days. Maybe you consume too much online information and it's playing havoc with your inner calm? Maybe you watch the news before you go to bed which leaves your brain frazzled and your inner anger raging? Or maybe you're online browsing websites, letting that bright screen infiltrate your sleepy eyes. If any of this rings bells, make the change.

How we perceive the constant circus that plays out around us is also pertinent to feeling calm. If we only see the negative and have no time for the positive we will more than likely attract more in. If we can only see the lacking in others we will never see the good in ourselves. If we think the grass is always greener we will never be content with where we are or end up. We all have to view this constant information from a calm spot inside and know that we can take it on board if we wish to, then act with a compassionate heart and open mind. We can be proactive, peaceful, disinterested, engaged, compassionate, indifferent, loving or inspired. The choice is yours. There are many options as to how we see the world. It isn't necessarily easy or second nature to us, but we can all try to tweak our natural inclinations. We might not be able to ignore the constant noise of the outside world but we can certainly hear many different tones if we listen hard enough.

Let it All Happen Naturally

HELLO TO . . . RUSSELL

Russell Brand needs very little introduction, as you will all be familiar with his incredible quick-witted and capacious vocabulary, self-deprecating tendencies and free-flowing locks. He has been on our screens and radios for nearly two decades and has had gargantuan levels of success, which of course in his line of work brings fame. I have known Russell on and off over the years and have always been intrigued as to how he has kept such a cool head whilst being in the centre of continuous outside judgment and assumption. When in the audience of his 2010 stand-up show I greatly admired how he turned particular career lows into a moment of self-deprecating humour. He has a remarkable way of making fun of himself and the events that surround his life and mines the humour out of it all. Everyone has an opinion about him yet he remains calm and focused on what he loves to do and wants to achieve. I find this massively inspirational, as viewing his own focus from afar makes me want to care even less about others' opinions, which in turn is very freeing and calming! Also, he is bloody clever . . . so . . .

F: Hello Russell. How calm would you say you are today in comparison to in your twenties and thirties?

R: Compared to that maniac I'm as serene as Jesus. Which is ironic because in my twenties and thirties I thought I was Jesus.

F: You've experienced fame to an extreme extent. Does being in the epicentre of public furore make for a chaotic existence?

R: When you take it seriously and allow it to form your identity and nourish your self-worth, which I did, it does.

F: How do you cope with outside opinion? Does it ever affect you in a negative way?

R: Yes it does, which I think is natural. We are social animals and without other people, who are we? The important thing is to have a source of nutrition that is not controlled by others.

F: You've taken breaks from social media but now use it to seemingly have fun (singing to your dog Bear) and also to talk about subjects you're very passionate about. Do you enjoy that public transaction?

R: I am a performer, I love to show off and I love to help people (when I'm not feeling self-obsessed) so social media, used wisely, can be great.

F: How do you keep calm when everyone else seems to be kicking up a fuss about your own narrative?

R: By recognising that what other people think about me is none of my business. This sense of independence is easier to achieve when I feel inwardly connected and I am not looking to external resources for validation.

F: Why do you think others get so involved in a story that has nothing to do with them directly?

R: Gossip as a means to understand your place in a social system is a vital tool. This tool has been overused and overwrought in order to keep people focused on consuming rather than inner evolution. If people feel at ease they buy less stuff.

F: Finally, Russell, what does calm mean to you?

R: Calm means being happy where I am, with who I am and who I'm with.

F: THANKS for your time and energy!

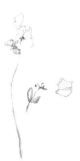

PROGRAMMED FROM BIRTH

We are massively programmed from birth to feel FEAR.

'Be careful little one, don't climb so high up that tree, it's dangerous.'

'Don't drink too much of that, it'll rot your teeth and they'll all fall out.'

'Stop jumping on the bed, you might fall off and hit your head.'

We are warned from the get go. Then at school we are taught to achieve otherwise we'll fail in the future. More fear. As teenagers when we are crossing the threshold into adulthood we are warned to not get pregnant, to not stay out too late on our own, to not waste time. Then as adults we are scared into parenting with mittens on. We are fed stories that make us feel terrified about our kids not getting enough nutritious foods, watching too much TV, not reaching milestones. A lot of it is fear and panic rather than hope and a calm approach.

So how do we find HOPE amid this cyclone of worry? It can feel very tough at times as we have been programmed for so many years to be this way. If you are passionate and committed to a particular religion this usually offers some respite from the onslaught of panic because you have trust in something or someone else more powerful than the mortal world. If you are not religious it can feel alien to trust anything other than what we read online, in papers or hear from others. The outside world has a huge impact on our level of fear and stress. We have been subconsciously taught that it is perhaps naive or fluffy to be hopeful.

I was born optimistic and carried on this way until into my twenties. Although I had a mother who was a bit of a worrier, like many others out there, I managed to hold on to the sunny side of life for a long time. After some of life's trickier patches my optimism was dampened and trodden upon and I haven't been able to get fully back into the swing of sunshine surfing since. I'm sure I'll get there but certain speed bumps in the road threw me right off track. I'm sad about this as I used to feel a lot calmer when 'optimism' was my middle name. I could get myself out of a tricky or limiting situation by believing there was something better. Due to my emphatic, hopeful visions, there usually was another option and I was always very open to finding it.

Being hopeful is now something that I work on daily. Having hope is not only a joy but very calming. If you truly believe and have trust in life, stress has to take a back seat and watch in awe as you calm your every cell and overactive mind by simply knowing that everything will be okay. Panic feels suffocated with hope around, which makes for a much calmer approach to the fear and noise around us. We all have a right to think like this and shouldn't feel foolish for doing so. We hear so much about the awful, catastrophic and grim things happening to planet Earth that we could be led to believe there is no good out there at all. But what about all the miracles that don't get reported? People who have been cured of illnesses they thought would kill them. Babies born to the supposedly infertile. Love found in desperate barren times. Peace reached after trauma. They do exist beyong the negative. The connection between us and miracles happening is 'hope'. It's one small word that builds a bridge between us struggling humans and total joy. I have found personally that if I focus on my dreams, fantasies and wishes, and reinforce them with solid 'hope', I feel a little calmer in believing they might just come true, or at least I'll have fun finding out if they do.

REGRETS AND 'WRONG' DECISIONS

When someone else tells you you've made the wrong decision, how much of this opinion should be taken on board? This is another tricky mountain to climb when applying the omnipresent buzz of the OUTSIDE world to our own story. Have you ever committed to one idea then been told it was the wrong one? A bad choice, a chancy decision or poor option? I certainly have! We have been taught since we were little that there are good paths to choose and also bad ones, but how much importance should we place on this outside opinion? When we are confronted with an opinion that differs from our own it can feel near impossible to not panic about our choices. Calm evaporates in a second and we are left feeling like we have made a mistake.

Recently I turned a job down as I already had family plans that day, which felt far more important to me to stick to. Some around me vehemently voiced that I had made the 'wrong' decision. I still felt that my priorities were 'right' for me but I'd be lying if I said I didn't waver for a second. I felt edgy all day as a part of me believed that I had made a mistake. I started to mistrust my own instinct. Retrospectively, I know I made the right choice for me but it's so tricky to ignore the voices and advice of others around us.

Sometimes we can look back and see that possibly we may have done things a little differently and we label these moments as mistakes. Mistakes are inevitable in life and they're also there for a reason. They create the most fertile ground in which lessons grow and have the ability to establish as seminal moments in life. Game changers, if you will! From these moments can spring new directions, a chance to start again and take a fresh perspective on all that has gone before.

It's very hard not to look back at times that we see as faulty or mistaken and not feel regret. Regrets are such a waste of time, and although I have a long list of them, I know deep down they are pointless and draining. We need to accept the paths we have taken and the roads we have trodden and try to look for the silver lining even if the outcome isn't what we want. If we know we listened too much to the outside chatter and too little to our inner dialogue and instinct, readdress this moment and learn from it, rather than beat yourself up for 'getting it wrong'. Most of the time when we feel we've made a mistake it's because we have made a decision based on fear. It could be a fear of what others will think, a fear of how we'll match up to others, or a fear of being judged. Sure, take on advice and support from others, but go with your gut always. If your gut gives you an answer, I believe you have to honour it and see where it might lead you. If we honour these moments and decisions it stops us feeling regret. If we know we have followed our gut, even if tonnes of people say you've got it wrong, you'll know deep down that you've got it bang on! You've made a decision based on instinct and from a calm place.

If things feel too cloudy and everyone's opinions have blurred your own instinct, sit on it. Go to bed and think on it again the next day, or sit quietly and try to clear your head from the outside world and see what pops up for you. The answer is usually in there somewhere if we give ourselves enough space to allow that gut feeling to surface. This way we can make clear, concise and definite decisions in a calm way.

We know the non-stop buzz of energy on planet Earth will continue to hum on and more than likely grow in volume. We know that each ticking second of the day globally contains happiness, sorrow, anger, injustice, revelation and every other possible emotion and outcome. We can't change any of it but we can stand strong in our own opinions from a peaceful place and we can view all of the noise from a grounded place. I guess we have to all attempt to stop comparing ourselves to everyone else and to stop feeling scared of what others are saying around us by firefighting it with hope and listening to our own instinct as much as we can. The huge task of staying calm in a modern world will forever perplex most of us, but if we are viewing, digesting and acting from a wholehearted place we can all hope to experience some calm along the way.

Summary

LOOK UP.

Put the phone down! Never forget to appreciate all the wonderful things around you.

PINCH OF SALT.

Don't believe everything you see on social media – we all know that but need reminding of it.

CHOOSE HOPE.

Don't let the world's negativity get to you; positive leads to calm and vice versa.

WHAT DOES CALM AND THE OUTSIDE WORLD LOOK LIKE TO YOU?

Write one word or draw a picture here that sums it up.

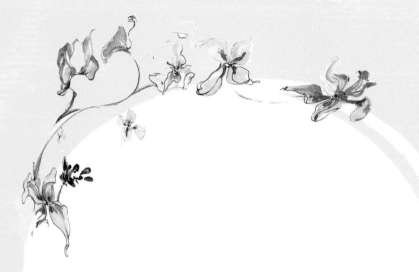
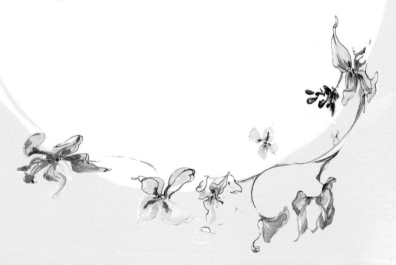

CALM

MY CALM IS...

My kids eating well at meal times

Feeling healthy and vibrant

Peeking in on my kids when they're asleep

Listening to chilled music on a hot evening

Reading my kids books at night time

My husband's smile

Being in a crowd at a festival. It is all about getting lost in the music and not about anyone around me

An early night

My dad's hugs

My mum's advice

My kids waking up any time after 6:30a.m.! A lie in!

My husband in the bed next to me (when he isn't snoring)

Watching a comedy with my step-kids

Baking cakes

Yoga. Every time. Total sanity-inducing calm

Running by the River Thames

Painting portraits of people I love

Toes in the sand

A decent sunset

The smell of the sea

Stargazing

Writing. Words, thoughts, stories

A good book in the bath

Being on time

Listening. To others. To the noises around me

Being cosy inside when it's bucketing down outside

When one of our cats sits on my lap

Rooibos tea with honey in it

Hanging out with my friend Lolly. Chatter and laughter

Drawing pictures with a black biro

Riding my bike through the park

Lying on the grass and looking at the sky

Lying in a hammock. This one doesn't happen enough

Lying anywhere

Sitting in the HIVE at Kew Gardens

The smell of incense

Remembering to be hopeful.

Calm, I'm learning more and more about your potency every day. I used to think you were terribly boring and only for the elite or old. How wrong I was. I veered so far from your cosy arms and wandered into so much stress and chaos, constantly pushing my own boundaries to see how hardy I was. I realise now that I could have achieved most of what I have, met as many brilliant people as I have and loved as much as I have, without all the anarchy and stress. It was mainly a waste of energy. At times my inner fire and angst helped propel me somewhat but I still believe I could have used my tenacious side in a calmer way and still had the experiences I have had. Perhaps I had to go to some lengths in the opposite direction to truly understand how much I need you.

I've got so much better at listening to your soothing tones and grounded words. I love that when I'm completely in touch with you I can make decisions with clarity, stride through tricky situations with a little more confidence and waste a lot less energy on the unnecessary. I have learned to embrace you when you are glowing strong, and I know I can lean on you and trust in you fully. I have witnessed so many around me do the same and breeze through situations with ease that I would have perhaps previously have slogged through ungraciously. I love that you find me in unexpected pockets of time and allow me to relax into a new pace that rejuvenates and heals. With your comfort and grounding I know I can patch up old wounds, find solace in others and stop to just BE when I feel the need. I have also worked out that it's a complete myth that you can't get much done when you're around. You're so not purely for the carefree, enlightened souls out there; you're for the vivacious, scatty, adventurous and tenacious and you work so well with these attributes, too. You can actually accelerate the power behind the more high-octane sides of life, by allowing consideration and clarity to run the show. Stress and anxiety end up slowing down a lot of action in life as we get stuck and become afraid, whereas you allow us to stride forward purposefully but without ego or inauthenticity getting in the way. Never again will I think of you as boring. I will look for you in busy parties, packed Tube stations, anarchic kids' parties and rushy school runs and know that you're in there somewhere. I'll also so look forward to getting to know you that bit better when I put my mind to it. On my yoga mat, in a good book, in meditation and in listening to my gut.

Thank you, Calm, you're really bloody lovely!

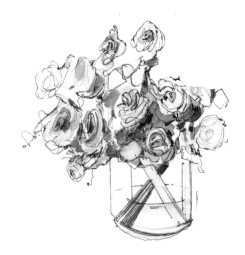

THANK YOUS

There are few better ways to feel CALM than saying 'thank you' to people who you adore, so here goes:

First up, a huge CALM thank you to Amanda Harris from Orion for giving me the nudge to write another book. I am forever grateful that you have given me such time and freedom to write down whatever is lurking in my head. Also a huge thank you to Emily Barrett from Orion for receiving many a late night email containing hundreds of questions and worries about what is buzzing around in my head. Thanks for the guidance and encouragement during our many edits. Cake will be sent to the Orion offices imminently.

Thank you to Holly Bott and Sophie Melia from James Grant media group for a plethora of constant good deeds. You are the ultimate gang to get a girl through writing a book. Thanks for taming my insecurities, helping me organise my time and for the mutual appreciation of the old-school Adidas tracksuit.

Thank you to Rowan Lawton of Furniss Lawton for having an encyclopedic literary knowledge and a mutual love of cakes. Your advice and wisdom on all things 'book' are invaluable to me and my writing. Your encouragement and advice has helped in so many ways.

Thanks to Abi Hartshorne at HART STUDIO for making CALM look so gorgeous and well . . . CALM. The colour palette, placement of illustrations and all-round aesthetic feels spot on. Thank you Jessica May Underwood you beautiful, talented, pixie of a person for your outstanding watercolour illustrations in the book. I am

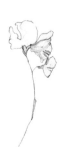

always in awe of your skill and imagination. Your delicate touch marries perfectly with my harsher biro drawings, complementing my words and creating joy all round.

Thank you to my lovely husband Jesse and my kids and step-kids, Arthur, Lola, Rex and Honey for giving me time and space in the evenings to sit hunched over my laptop until my eyelids start to burn. You are a constant joy to me and bring me equal measures of chaos and calm to keep me learning. Thanks to my family and friends who are always at the end of the phone to hear my wobbles and worries and to douse me in CALM. I only hope I offer you the same back. If not, at least I make a mean carrot cake when you come round to the house.

Love and peace always.

ABOUT THE AUTHOR

Fearne has been on our screens presenting live TV since the age of 15 when she was spotted by ITV's Disney Club. She is a team captain on 'Celebrity Juice' and her other programmes include 'The BBC Music Awards,' 'Top of the Pops' with Reggie Yates, 'Children in Need Rocks' with Chris Evans and live broadcasts from both the Royal Wedding and Princess Diana concert for BBC. In 2005 she joined Radio 1 where she spent 10 years, initially co-hosting morning shows with Reggie Yates, and then moving onto the UK Top 40 show before taking over the prestigious weekday morning slot in 2009. The show attracted over 4 million listeners and in 2012 she won a Sony Gold Award for the show. Most recently Fearne has turned her attention to her creative side, working in collaboration with Cath Kidston and designing a children's clothing range with Mini Club for Boots.

With many millions of followers on social media, she is ranked amongst the world's 250 most influential tweeters. Fearne lives in London with her family.

OTHER TITLES
BY FEARNE

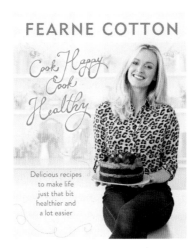

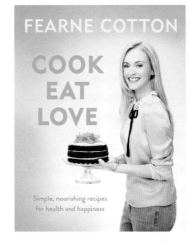

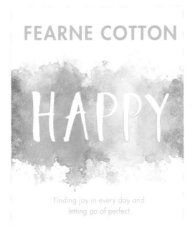

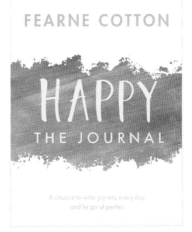